Nourish Your Self Whole

Nourish

Your Self Whole

A GUIDE TO THE CORE DIETARY PILLARS,
WITH ACHIEVABLE STEPS FOR VIBRANT HEALTH
Plus, meaningful lifestyle tips to enrich your whole self

by Matthew Albracht

Cover photo by: Larisa Blinova

KEEP INFORMED!

JOIN MATTHEW'S EMAIL LIST

For many free ongoing health and wellness updates and tips, please join Matthew's email list.

Visit: www.NourishYourSelfWhole.com

Follow him on:
Facebook: www.facebook.com/MatthewAlbracht
Twitter: www.twitter.com/MatthewAlbracht
Instagram: www.instagram.com/MatthewAlbracht

My inspiration to write this book was in large part my family and friends. I cherish my loved ones, my community. I hope the information within feeds and nourishes you as you have me. May all of us live healthier, happier and longer lives— and celebrate many more good times together!

Table of Contents

Preface

Dear Friend,
I feel honored and touched that you are diving into this world of health and wellness with me.

I felt inspired to write this book because I wanted to capture the most essential elements that helped me heal in my own life, and share them with loved ones or anyone else who might feel the pull to read and learn. This book reflects years of careful research and applied practice. In addition to my own firsthand experience of the benefits described within and my training as a health coach, I've relied on well-respected researchers and other highly qualified experts to help inform the pillars and pointers I'm sharing in this book.

I wrestled with the pros and cons of writing a full book. I thought through why it was needed when there are so many other good resources out there on these topics—many of which I have read. After careful thought, I decided to move forward for the following reasons.

Most respectable books out there on the topic go pretty deep into all the nuances of what it takes to eat and live well. I really appreciate reading all the layers of data and information, it's something that gets me excited. I want to overturn every stone and really understand the depths of an issue I care about. Nutrition is definitely one of those areas, as are the other lifestyle improvements I delve into.

But here, I wanted to home in on the most highly leveraged steps, that would have the most impact to best maximize your valuable time and energy, without getting too deep into the weeds that I think many books get into.

As I became a certified health coach, which I do part time amidst other work in the social change arenas, I learned quickly that many people don't have the time or often the interest in going so deep. They just want the basics to give them enough information to move forward into a healthier life, of feeling better, with as much ease as possible. That became the driving force in my motivation and decision to write this book: to distill down the basics, specifically the most important steps that anyone could and should take to live more healthily—to provide more of the essentials that everyone needs to take on to get to significant improvements and a solid baseline of wellness. And I think I've done it. I certainly hope I have. I distilled it down into four basic pillars of good nutrition.

I have worked hard to provide you with information that is as simple and straightforward as possible without spending an inordinate amount of time on the intricacies of the science behind the principles or the myriad ways you can achieve improved health. Where I feel it's needed, I go deeper, but I wanted to create something a little different than most of the other "diet and wellness" books out there. My central goal is to get you enough facts, information, and practical tips to help you follow these health practices as easily as possible. Again, I have tried to keep the focus on the most highly leveraged steps; that is, the ones that will have the greatest impact on your good health. And if I go too deep into the weeds for you, I've tried to structure the information in a way that you can skip forward if you feel ready. Read and use this book in whatever way best meets your needs! It doesn't have to be read in order. The table of contents should be particularly helpful as it is very detailed by design, and you can jump to the sections that most inspire you or that you want delve more deeply into. I would advise you to read at least the basic intro points about each pillar, so you know enough to make solid choices.

In the introduction, I set the context for why a healthy lifestyle is important. I review the benefits and explore how they will help your whole body feel better. There are some important points there, but if you are feeling ready to get to the fundamentals, feel free to skim the introduction for relevant information and then jump right into the four pillars.

The first part of this book focuses on four pillars, the most important nutritional steps you can take. These are the foundation for any good diet. Tackling them alone will bring you many great health benefits, and will give you the most bang for your buck when it comes to spending your time and energy efficiently. Every step you take, even if only small initial ones, will have an impact.

In order to make all the key nutritional information easier to remember and work with, you can also download a handy **Printable Cheat Sheet Shopping List** I created just for readers of this book—with key lists and tips that I included within my tips sections from each of the four pillars. Just print it out to take with you, or save the .pdf to your smartphone so you always have it. Visit: www.nourishyourselfwhole.com/printable-cheat-sheet

The last third of the book focuses on additional food, lifestyle and environmental factors that will take you even farther down the road to vibrant health. These factors branch out in many directions, including managing stress, minimizing environmental toxins, and other relevant areas-- with tips and information that will help you fine-tune and improve your overall wellness.

There are many fantastic experts working in the health and wellness field. In fact, I have a list of my own favorite books, podcasts, expert websites, and so on at the end of this book. In this book, including the resource list, I talk a lot about Functional Medicine practitioners (who are typically M.D.s). If you are unfamiliar with the term, *Functional Medicine* is a systems biology–based approach to identifying and addressing the root causes of disease.

Even if you are a staunch believer in traditional Western medicine, Functional Medicine support can be a great supplement to your standard annual physical and blood work. I encourage you to further explore any or all of the additional resources that pique your interest. The creators of these resources are the top experts in their respective fields, providing you with a plethora of detailed information on how to fine-tune your health down to practically every micro-detail.

Thanks for taking this little journey with me into increased health and wellness for yourself. Again, I've done my best to make this accessible and full of useful tips for living a healthier and more vibrant life. I genuinely hope that the information within nourishes your life in some tangible ways. My own journey through the process of researching and writing has certainly helped deepen and clarify my own self-care practices. I've learned a lot about myself through it and feel like a better and happier man because of it.

I hope this book meets or even exceeds your expectations. Either way, please let me know how you feel about it. Any feedback you give could help me improve future editions. (info@nourishyourselfwhole.com)

Finally, since I wrote this book with the novice in mind, I decided not to cite every single point of science in the book. I did however create a bibliography that includes some of the key research on the claims within, which you can read if you are like me and want to geek out or carefully review some of the science.

All the best,

Matthew Albracht

January 18, 2021

P.S. As I'm finishing up edits on this book, we are in the throes of the Coronavirus COVID-19 global pandemic. It's certainly a wild moment in human history. I hope everyone is taking good care as it's likely this will be a challenge for the long haul. The good news about this book is that everything in it will be helpful in getting your body and mind in healthier shape to deal with this, or any virus or illness that might come along.

What we know for sure is that those who are in the best overall health fare the best when challenged with this virus or most any other illness. The food pillars I discuss will all be a solid support in helping you get into much better health, and boost and strengthen your immune system unlike what almost anything else can.

I would also encourage you to put special attention on the last third of this book as well, that deals with many additional lifestyle pillars that can help boost our bodies and minds. Whether it's emotional support tools for dealing with the stressors this pandemic is bringing up, tips for reducing environmental toxins that tax our systems, getting into better physical shape, etc., I've presented a nice overview of resources and ideas on many areas that will help you better navigate this moment (and your whole life).

This can be a time that derails us or a time that deepens our commitments to better personal and societal health that can make us all far more resilient for the long haul. I choose the later and am doubling down myself to get in even better mental and physical health. Hope you will join me.

A couple of additional side notes: My editor made an astute point that I use the words "challenge" or "issue" frequently in this book, in lieu of other more traditionally used words and phrases like "problem," or "condition," etc., and that it might be helpful to share early on in the book why I'm making that choice. I believe that many of the "issues" or "challenges" we face are not insurmountable obstacles, but in fact can be opportunities to overcome and transform with the right positive influences. And that's all part of life, we always have challenges to face and move through, it builds stronger character and wisdom, or at least it can. Words like "problem" are so loaded and negative in my estimation, so I try to avoid. It's both a practical and philosophical choice I'm making, as I don't want to limit possibility by reinforcing old negative patterns of thinking and beliefs, and instead focus my language to try and help motivate.

Finally, I will be mentioning some specialty diets, including the Paleo Diet or Ancestral Diet as it's sometimes referred, which is the diet I mainly adhere to. In a nutshell, the paleo diet is an anti-inflammatory diet that has looked at the kinds of foods our ancestors have eaten for thousands of years (before modern times), and built their ideas around how we evolved to eat. There is a lot of wisdom in this approach as it is how our bodies adapted to eat. I don't use this diet as my primary template in this book, I instead am using broader and more universal principles and distilling down the most important keys. That being said, everything I espouse is also mostly a part of the Paleo diet, and if you are looking to go more in depth after you finish this book, I'd suggest checking this diet out. (There is not one official version, many folks work in the field. You can look at my recourses section at end of book for my favorites.)

Quick Glance Overview:
The Four Most Important Pillars to Good Health

Foundational Pillar 1: **Eat a Whole Foods Diet.** We did not evolve eating the chemically laced and overly processed foods that line much of our grocery shelves. The additives and preservatives work against our thriving health in a myriad of ways and can destroy good "probiotic" gut bacteria. If there are more than five ingredients listed on the label and/or you can't pronounce them or would need a translation, then a good rule of thumb is to skip it! This pillar underlies all the rest. You'll find that if you follow the other three pillars below, there aren't many highly processed foods you should or would want to indulge much in anyway.

Pillar 2: **Reduce Sugar and Refined Carbs** – We'll explore why you should reduce your intake of refined sugars and simple carbohydrates. Too much sugar is highly inflammatory in the body and is a hot bed for diabetes, heart disease, and cancer. It can disrupt healthy functioning of insulin and other important hormones, and can cause weight gain by triggering the body to store fat, along with a whole host of other troubling consequences. In fact, high fructose corn syrup, the main sweetener in sugary soda and many other processed foods, is now believed to be one of the top disease creators on the planet.

Highly processed grains, especially refined (or "white") flours, quickly turn into sugar in your bloodstream as well, so they should be kept to a minimum.

Pillar 3: **Eat Good Fats, Ditch Bad Fats** – You've probably heard by now that there are good and bad dietary fats. We will look at why you should delight in eating plenty of healthy and satiating fats. These can include: extra virgin olive oil, avocado oil, coconut oil (all cold-pressed); and for non-vegetarians/vegans, ghee, high-quality fish oil, and grass-fed animal fats. These kinds of healthy fats offer critical nutrients. They are often anti-inflammatory and help fuel your body more sustainably than sugar.

Most of us aren't actually getting enough good fat, so add a little butter back to those sautéed vegetables! We'll also explore why you should eliminate bad, inflammatory fats, which we are getting far too much of in our modern diets, but can be a major contributor to cancer and heart disease, to name a few. These include easily oxidized industrial oils from vegetable seeds like canola, soy, corn, safflower, sunflower, and so on. (Yes, I know, we've been told over the last few decades that they are better than whole food based unrefined fats, but they are not). It's also critical to strictly avoid all hydrogenated and trans fats, but beware—they are hiding out in all kinds of processed foods. The good news is that you can be quite liberal with how much healthy fat you are eating, swap it out for the refined carbs and sugars. Be decadent!

Pillar 4: **Indulge in a Rainbow of Vegetables (and a Bit of Fruit): Vitamins, Minerals, Antioxidants, Phytonutrients and Fiber** – Eat as many vegetables as you can possibly consume each day. Six to ten servings a day are a good target. Fruits can be important, too; just keep them on the modest side. They are loaded with sugar. Fruit should be kept to one to two servings a day, if even that, depending on how well your body can balance its blood sugar (more on this inside).

Delight in as many colors and varieties of vegetables and fruits as you can. When it comes to produce, the individual colors of the rainbow contain different phytonutrients that are critical for our bodies' optimal function. The vast array of nutrients all contribute to a vibrantly functioning body and are especially crucial in keeping disease-causing stimuli (like inflammation) at bay. They are the best antidote to wrangling free radicals in your body, which are a primary cause of cancer. So, eat up!

Nourish Your Self Whole

Introduction:

What you put on your fork is the most important thing you do every day. It influences your capacity to live a rich, energetic, connected, soulful life—a life in which you have the energy to care for yourself, to love your friends and family, to help your neighbor, to fully show up for your work in the world, and to live your dreams. If you enjoy real, whole, fresh foods that you cook using real ingredients, you are positively affecting everything around you. Simply put: Food is the doorway to living well and loving well— and to fixing much of what's wrong with our world.
— Dr. Mark Hyman,
Food: What the Heck Should I Eat?

Are you feeling like your body is struggling more and more to serve you in the way it once did? Are you experiencing any of the following:

- *Feeling run-down more often than you'd like or than you feel that you should?*
- *Feeling foggy-headed and/or desperate for a nap every day, especially after that lunchtime sandwich?*
- *Missing the energy you had in your younger years?*
- *Feeling frustrated by creaky, stiff joints and muscles that seem to be growing rapidly worse with age?*
- *Needing but are having a hard time getting quality sleep?*
- *Feeling hunger pangs just an hour or two after eating your granola for breakfast or sandwich for lunch?*
- *Having challenges shedding the extra weight that has crept slowly upon your frame over the years?*
- *Getting diagnosed with potentially serious health challenges?*
- *With the way things are going, are you feeling concerned that you might be barreling toward a challenging last leg of your life, when it arrives?*

These questions represent just some of the scenarios of the slow decline in health and the related challenges that many of us face. Most of us incorrectly accept them as something inevitable and irreversible as we age. We put the blame on the good or bad luck we inherited through our gene pool. Too many of us are buying into these overly simplistic, often false ideas. They have little basis in the leading-edge science, which now shows that proper nutrition and lifestyle habits are the overwhelmingly predominant drivers of our body's proper functioning and our overall health and can even turn around entrenched health challenges. (Environmental factors also play a key role.)

Healthy food and lifestyle choices are more than virtuous practices. They are often the magic key to keeping our body running in its optimal and precision-tuned natural state of wellness. The unhealthy choices we make are frequently the driving force behind our undue degradation, far more than most people realize. Of course, we are going to decline with age, but it doesn't necessarily have to be at the pace or severity with which many of us are currently declining.

The encouraging news that I'm excited to share with you in this book is that vibrant and enlivening health are well within reach for most people. Good food is medicine. Weaving the nutritional pillars in this book into your life can help create substantial healing for your body and get you back into the shape in which you can thrive. This will inevitably lead to a more fulfilling and energetic life. And, I believe, it's one of the ultimate acts of self-love.

There are many nutrition and lifestyle influences we can all pursue to achieve optimal wellness. **The four pillars highlighted within these pages are your best bet when it comes to creating good health, vitality, and a more fulfilling life.** Just as physical pillars hold up a building, these four pillars will support your fundamental health and lead you to inspiring results. They are in line with the most up-to-date research, and with nutritional experts who have evidence of success from their own applied practice working with tens of thousands of patients. I too have seen these principles work in my own life and through my nutritional coaching & education practice time and time again. (The last section of the book will also discuss some important lifestyle and environmental supports that will add even more benefit should you choose to take some of it on.)

The Overall Health Benefits of This Plan

These pillars can help you:
- Prevent and, in many cases, reverse disease
- Generate more energy and vitality
- Improve mood
- **Lose unwanted weight** without worrying much about calories (eat plenty of the good stuff!)
- Improve blood sugar and cholesterol
- Shed longstanding body aches and pains
- Clear up foggy-headedness
- Create vibrant skin
- Experience better sleep
- And more…

Pursuing the course of action spelled out in this book will form a solid foundation for anyone seeking a better quality of life. It will almost certainly help you realize noticeably positive results. While the pillars are not the only things you can do for better health, they are at the top of the list.

I'll take you step by step through how you can integrate these changes into your current eating habits with relative ease, while creating maximal results. Even those of you juggling a "crazy busy" modern life can implement pieces of the plan as you are able and start to improve. Every step you take, even the small ones, will make a difference. It will be a positive change away from the Standard American Diet (or as many call it, the "SAD" diet), into a more healthy and nutrient dense diet that focuses on eating delicious, fresh whole foods that can help supercharge a vibrant life.

The most important thing to keep in mind is that **all four of the pillars work in powerful concert with one another**. Each supports the other in crucial ways that will reveal themselves as you read through the book. That doesn't mean you have to be at 100% compliance in every one to get benefits, every step you take will help, but the further along you push the envelope into each of the pillar's guidelines, the more benefit you'll obviously see.

This is NOT a deprivation "diet." It's a lifestyle eating shift that is full of genuinely amazing food. We will go through some **healthy and delicious alternatives** to the "comfort foods" that you might feel the most resistant to let go of. Most "diets" fail when they require participants to deprive themselves of tasty and needed energy-producing foods that are essential for both nourishment and satisfaction.

Moderation can certainly be important around the habits that do not contribute to our flourishing health. While you might eat less of the treats and foods you are used to, depending on what kinds of foods you are eating now, you will find very hearty and satisfying alternatives to the not so great stuff. In fact you'll likely find that you won't need to eat as much when you are giving your body the deep nourishment it needs. That is the REALLY good news.

A long-term healthy diet is not one of severe limitations. In fact, it includes a host of hearty foods that will leave you feeling satiated and more than content. You shouldn't feel as if you are hungry all the time. If you are, then you are likely not doing it right!

When I started my own health journey, the most surprising thing I learned was that I could really eat as much food as I wanted and needed. I just switched to the right stuff: very tasty and satisfying alternatives. In fact, nowadays when friends and family come over for a meal I prepare, they are almost always shocked I eat such rich and yummy foods and still maintain a slim figure. (Not to mention my positive lab health markers and indicators).

A typical meal might be roasted wild salmon served with a hearty butter, sage, and white balsamic reduction. On the side could be some sweet potatoes roasted in a little avocado oil, along with zucchini and kale sautéed in coconut oil and a mixed green salad full of colorful additions. Maybe even an almond or cassava-flour chocolate chip cookie for an occasional treat. (Note: many folks can't even tell these are not made from traditional wheat-based flour, they are sooo good).

Let's get real for a minute. You might think you can't live without unfavorable foods like white rice or cheap, starchy bread, but when you get used to the textures and deep flavors of whole foods of good quality, your body systems and your taste buds will change for the better. You will find the subtleties of good food to be more than just satiating and satisfying. I, for one, have more than adjusted to this new way of eating. Being on the other side of these changes, I now enjoy food even more than I did before. The more complex and nuanced flavors now have space on my tongue to dance around a bit and to feel appreciated. Before, they were overwhelmed by the hyper-flavorings of processed foods—intense sweeteners, fake seasonings, or cheap fats and grains designed to act like a nuclear explosion on the tongue (and in the body). Junk foods I once found tasty or had intense cravings for now often overwhelm me and seem cheap and hollow. My taste buds and body's desires have transformed. There is a whole new world of delightful flavors and experiences to be had with food when you give yourself over to quality.

Following these four pillars can also help you balance your weight without having to focus too much on counting calories. Getting your body back in balance and eating the nutrient-dense foods your body desperately needs will often do the trick when it comes to weight management. Not only does the research point to this, I've also seen it happen many times to folks I've worked with, not to mention my own personal experience.

I honestly don't think much about how many calories I'm eating in a meal anymore. But I'm not one of those people who is just naturally rail thin. When I started this dietary shift, I quickly lost close to twenty pounds that I'd slowly collected over the years. My intense cravings have significantly balanced out as I've made the shifts that I describe within these pillars.

As you will read, I along with many health experts believe we've been hoodwinked by some of the "healthy eating" advice pushed out in recent decades. The foods that have been demonized, like healthy fats for example, are actually some of the most nourishing and balancing nutrients. When I was growing up in the eighties, we were told that fat of almost any kind was the work of the devil. I thought that my slow weight gain was surely because of the robust doses of olive oil I'd started to use more frequently, imagine my surprise when I learned it was actually all those refined carbs I was indulging in! Thankfully the facts are starting to get out and public perceptions are changing.

Before I became trained in Functional Nutrition, I had heard broadly about some of the enclosed recommendations. Generally speaking, I knew the benefits of and tried as much as I thought I could to eat a relatively healthy, mostly organic, whole-foods diet. However, I didn't comprehend the depth of the impact I could make on my own health until I started taking on these pillars for myself. Once I started to dig in and truly make changes, my health shifted radically for the better. The results were beyond what I could have imagined. I'll share more as we move on about my own health journey as it relates to this.

Be brave. This dietary lifestyle shift is not only worth it; it's also not that hard.

For some of you, the four dietary pillars within these pages may initially seem daunting. Meanwhile, others may already be on the path to some degree.

I know when I started my health journey, I thought some of the suggested shifts seemed downright intimidating! In particular, I thought I might never be able to make the shift away from my relatively high-carb diet. I LOVED my far-too-frequent pancakes and pastries. (I still have them sometimes, but with some healthier tricks I'll share later on.) A meal didn't seem like a meal without something bready or starchy. I thought I needed that feeling of having a lead brick in my belly to feel full!

Thankfully, scaling back on it all has not only made a tremendously positive impact on how I feel, but it was also not as hard as I thought it would be. My cravings for the junk faded significantly as I continued to eat healthy and delicious foods. I wouldn't have believed it at the time, but I now feel more steadily "full" and more satisfied than when I indulged in a million cheap carbs.

My Health Story

As I mentioned, I've been relatively conscious of my eating for the last twenty-five years. Back then, I ate what I thought was a pretty healthy diet. The good: I did my best to focus on whole foods, organic when possible, and shied away from too much processed and junk foods. (To varying degrees of success, but at least I knew what to do—or so I thought.)

But I, like many folks, had heard for much of my life that the real culprits for disease were cholesterol and fat. I have since learned that a plethora of current, and even past, scientific research indicates that this was likely never really the case; at least not as it has been advocated and lobbied for so many years. So, I largely avoided fats, except for assorted vegetable oils, which I used sparingly. I thought my organic hydrogenated vegetable-based margarine was to be applauded (*hint:* it's not). At some point, I'd heard olive oil was good, so I integrated a fair amount of that into my diet (*hint:* it's great).

I knew sugar wasn't a health food, but I naïvely thought sugar was only really dangerous if someone were diabetic. If one didn't have a family history of diabetes, it didn't seem like something to worry about, so I indulged my sweet tooth pretty regularly. I was doing better than the average American, but I loved my sodas at the movie theater and put extra syrup on my nearly every morning pancakes. (At least it was real maple syrup! At least the pancakes were gluten-free! Still loads of carbs, but I *thought* I was doing good...) An evening sweet treat was also not uncommon.

However, my favorite treats were of the salty variety: namely chips and salsa, which were deep-fried in hydrogenated, industrial vegetable seed oils, now known to wreak havoc on the body.

Breads and other grains, I'd been told, were great when made whole and with fiber, so I always made sure to eat (plenty of) high-fiber grains. As I said, I had to have them at pretty much every meal (see "pancakes with extra syrup" just mentioned). For common but not daily treats, I sure did love my pastries, such as scones, sticky buns, and the occasional donut. Mmm, mmm, mmm! (Okay, okay, I'm getting ahold of myself).

Anyway, other than those "few" bad habits, I THOUGHT I was doing fairly well with my eating.

The thing is, I felt sicker and sicker as the years progressed. I was more rundown and with overall devolving health. My gut was experiencing growing discomfort. My back started to hurt in my mid-twenties and deteriorated to the point where I couldn't sit for more than about ten minutes without wanting to squirm out of my skin in discomfort and pain.

By my early thirties, I was tired almost every afternoon, the kind of tired where I could visualize and desired laying on the floor (anywhere!) and immediately falling asleep. Throughout my twenties, I could sleep nine or ten hours, no sweat! By my forties, I had far too many short, restless, and fitful nights of sleep.

My joints started to get pretty creaky by my mid-thirties. I'd get out of bed and hear myself groan like my grandfather had every time he got out of his big recliner when I was growing up. "Uh-oh," I thought.

When I'd get my annual physical and blood work, my blood sugar was higher than it should have been, not quite prediabetes, but higher than ideal. This was happening pretty consistently, and I was getting concerned.

I started feeling foggy-headed most of the time. I couldn't focus very well, and my thinking often felt muddy. At the peak of my "brain fog," I remember dreading work meetings. It was hard needing to be "on" when I felt I could barely string a sentence together. I frequently cringed and apologized often for being so spacey. I am a fairly intelligent and motivated person, so it wasn't like I couldn't get anything done, but I was at a limited capacity. My memory had started to take a hit as well. Many days it felt like a big hit. In my teens and early twenties, I could remember everything! I took great pride in it. I felt disappointed to be losing that.

By my thirties, I was getting progressively more irritating skin issues, like odd, itchy rashes; a flaky scalp; frequent canker sores; and minor but annoying acne on my nose. (I did not think I was supposed to have acne in my thirties. Grrr!)

I was also getting a lot of inflammation in my mouth. Despite fairly rigorous brushing and flossing habits, my gums had tender spots, and they swelled and bled more as the years progressed. My dentist urged me to try all kinds of fancy treatments, like periodontal laser therapy, to keep me from getting gingivitis or having other long-term dental problems.

To complicate things even further, in my late teens, I had acquired an unfortunate intestinal auto-immune disease called *post-infectious IBS (irritable bowel syndrome)* from a really bad food-poisoning incident. This created much intestinal pain and discomfort as well as too many bathroom visits. These symptoms forced significant limits on my ability to function as normally as I would have liked to in my life. My IBS got progressively worse and ultimately became the impetus for me to make the more significant health shifts that led to the writing of this book.

As the years progressed, many of these issues occurred more frequently. Again, I was getting increasingly concerned.

I'd spent years seeing both traditional and alternative doctors, who ultimately had next to nothing to offer me for my increasing ailments. I was looking for any kind of quick fix, hoping there might be pills I could take to shift my health and improve my gut function (and all the other areas of challenge I was facing), to no avail. It all got bad enough finally that I surrendered. I wanted to make some fundamental changes and do the work I had long avoided, though had always suspected I probably had to do. In short, I decided to try a new track and a more rigorous nutritional regimen.

Soon after I made this deep, internal commitment, I dove into my research. I read quite a few books, tons of blogs, listened to countless hours of nutritional podcasts, and started to try things out. I tried more dietary healing strategies than most people even know exist. (It was certainly more than I'd heard of before!) The most important areas I stumbled upon were the interrelated worlds of Functional Medicine, anti-inflammatory and paleo/ancestral diets. I took on their lower carb, low-sugar, good-fats diets. When it started to work, it felt kind of like magic. Even within the first week, I felt much better in some key ways. I was clearer-headed, had more energy, and many of my aches and pains were noticeably lightening. After the first couple of months on my protocol, in some key ways, I felt like a different person.

One particularly vivid example I remember was when I went to the dentist for my annual exam, he was surprised by how much my gum inflammation had calmed down since just our last visit. When I explained what I'd been doing, he was one of the few medical professionals that totally understood the positive impact of my decision to give up sugar, go low carb, and swap out bad fats. He'd seen the negative impact on teeth and gum health for people who ate diets with too many of the inflammatory foods that I'd given up.

While my intestinal disease has proven a more challenging foil to resolve fully, I felt encouraged in comparison to how I had been feeling. Other than that, as the months progressed, every medical concern I mentioned above either significantly improved or fully went away. (Three cheers for clear skin!) It was a remarkable and encouraging shift, though I honestly couldn't believe it.

After all the years of looking for help, how had I not heard of this path and these particular nutritional tools to better health?

Shedding Some Pounds I Thought Were Here to Stay

My new health journey tackled another annoying challenge that I honestly hadn't considered when I started: my weight. Through my early twenties, I was as thin as a twig. By my early forties, though, I'd put on about twenty additional pounds from my leanest adult weight. At almost six feet tall, that twenty pounds wasn't classified as being terribly overweight, but I was not enjoying my growing gut or widening face. Oh, the vanity! (I knew it wasn't healthy, but I think I might have been more concerned with the growing gut.)

While I was in my "heavier" phase, I thought the real culprit was lack of exercise. While I exercised some, I thought it must not have been nearly enough. I supposed I'd have to really rev up the treadmill to boost my metabolism to the point where I could lose weight. I went through phases of consistent workouts, but never saw any real difference in weight. The one big food item I thought might be doing the most damage in terms of weight was that I used too much olive oil on my sautéed vegetables.

All of this thinking was fundamentally wrong. As you will learn in this book, extra weight isn't primarily from lack of physical activity—though that certainly does have some impact and is incredibly important to overall health—it is predominantly due to our food choices. And mine wasn't from too much fat, it was actually from too little and the wrong kinds (plus those excessive carbs and sugar!).

When I got on my new eating plan, the first and most surprising thing that happened was that the excess weight dropped off in about two months. I wasn't exercising any more than usual. Those twenty pounds have stayed off for years now! Maybe I was dense, but I had no idea this was possible primarily by shifting what I ate, rather than from either how much I ate or from intensive exercise.

A Shift in Mood

While the downward shift in my weight, and the other positive changes in my body that I just described were a more-than-pleasant surprise, the biggest surprise of all was a significant improvement in my mood and sense of emotional well-being.

I'd struggled with fairly intense anxiety since my teenage years, as well as various levels of moodiness. In my teens and early twenties there were even some dips into mild depression. All of these emotional issues challenged and taxed my sense of wellbeing.

I'd managed to make significant progress over the years, but some moodiness and anxiety still uncomfortably lingered. After about two or three months on my new diet, I started to feel a whole new sense of myself. There was a sense of calm that I hadn't felt since I was a carefree kid. It was marked and more than a bit surprising, but in a really good way. (I also started supplementing with vitamin B-12, which I found out I was low in through lab work, and can be related to mood issues.)

An important aside: to be clear, I've been doing committed psychological and spiritual growth work of numerous varieties for twenty-five years. All of this work has contributed amazingly and immeasurably towards my current sense of well-being and psychological and spiritual satisfaction. I'm not suggesting that this psycho/spiritual work on myself wasn't important for me, or that it isn't important for others. I'd made great strides even before my dietary changes and was feeling pretty happy with my progress and its trajectory.

In fact, I think the personal growth work I've done ultimately helped me love myself enough to get to the point of taking better nutritional care of myself. This is a real bottom line for so many of us: **Do we love ourselves enough to nourish and feed ourselves into a more vibrant and healthy physical being?** Or are some of us punishing ourselves, maybe even unconsciously, by feeding our worst habits and thought processes the worst foods we can give them? What parts of ourselves need more self-love and acceptance to allow for deeper healing? These kinds of questions might be important for you to explore as you begin to make some of these health changes. Later in the book, in the section entitled "Emotional Wellness, Stress Reduction and Healing Life's Traumas" I list a number of important modalities that could prove helpful in this front. I can't speak highly enough about the importance of investing time in addressing the psychological and emotional aspects of healing.

All of that being said, I also can't articulate strongly enough how surprised I was that my nutritional shifts contributed to my improved mental state. I had never heard much about nutrition's role in emotional well-being. I have now, of course. This concept is well understood in the Functional Medicine world, within which I'm immersed. In fact, there is a great deal of scientific literature on the role nutrition plays in our psychological well-being and it's receiving growing attention in the field.

For all of this positive physical and emotional progress, I was both deeply grateful and, I must admit, a bit disappointed that I'd learned about this important nutritional information so late in life. I was primarily grateful to have some encouraging relief and to have tools at my disposal that I could utilize in the long term, but I was frustrated about the decades I had spent searching so hard to find support to get physically better. If I'd had earlier guidance about how important nutrition is to health, and how to best wield a strategy to help myself, I might have been motivated enough to shift my diet years earlier.

It was more than disheartening to realize how ill-equipped our mainstream Western medical system is when it comes to dealing with chronic disease and the ailments we all face as a result of the "SAD" Standard American Diet and other environmental and lifestyle factors. Give a doctor a broken bone or an acute trauma, and they can fix you right up better than anyone, but Western medicine has little to offer the long, gestating challenges of chronic disease. This comes as no surprise when you learn that fewer than twenty percent of U.S. medical schools have a single required course in nutrition. I feel sad thinking of all the millions, more likely billions, who are unnecessarily suffering as a result. This is a huge part of why I am writing this book, to add my voice to the choir of advocates trying to get the word out. It's good news, but there is a lot of work to do!

I encourage you to be brave and bold in seeking the level of support that matches the overall health you'd like to feel. Having been through this and now living on the other side of it, I can assure you that it's worth it. I feel pretty great nowadays—not perfect, but in a much better flow when it comes to my health and vitality. Maybe you want to be strong and energetic enough to deeply engage with your kids or grandkids? Maybe the results on your scale or medical tests have you up at night with worries? Hopefully as you begin living a more healthful life, your experience will be positively similar to mine. I'll do my best to give you enough not only for a solid start, but also for you to believe that this is a worthy endeavor.

You are what you eat, for better or for worse.

Food is one of the most important influences on your overall health. Many of us erroneously chalk our health trajectory up to our genes, which is the biological equivalent of the luck of the draw. However, scientific research shows that about eighty-four percent of disease is actually determined by our *epigenetics*. Among other things, epigenetics can be heavily determined by nutritional, environmental, and lifestyle factors, with food being a top driver. This means that our health is not simply impacted by our innate or hereditary genes acting out. These epigenetic influences help decide which genes "express" themselves, that is, which ones are active or dormant, and ultimately impact our health. So for someone that eats fried fast food every day, they may have genes that are not ideal turned on and active, while another person eating a healthy diet may have those same dangerous genes remain in the "off" position. To sum it up, it's not just the genes you have in your DNA makeup, it's also how they are influenced and triggered by outside factors like food that influence your overall health.

As a culture, many of our health indicators are declining because of the impact of these negative epigenetic factors. Chronic disease rates are skyrocketing, and experts believe that changes in our collective food choices and culture-wide eating habits are some of the primary causes. This does not simply impact adults. **Chronic disease rates among children between 1994 and 2006 doubled!** This is a disturbing trend that cuts across the age spectrum, but especially seems to be growing with each new generation of children.

Why is this? Where food is concerned, diets high in sugar, refined carbs, and highly processed vegetable oils are not compatible with healthy genetic expression. That's right, genes don't function well on the heavy doses of these substances that most of us consume. The bad genes that we hear about in the news, such as Alzheimer's & breast cancer genes, don't necessarily cause their damage unless specific conditions activate them. When negative gene expressions are triggered, this in turn can cause many diseases and negative health conditions.

In other words, our genes aren't necessarily our destiny. The choices we make have a powerful influence, but the good news is that bad gene expressions have the potential to be reversed when controllable factors like food consumption are improved.

The bottom line for most of us is that there are too many irritants and toxins and not enough nutrients coming into the body. Nutrients can powerfully counteract the negative stimuli we are pummeled with each day, from air pollution to stress and poor food choices, among others. One of the most powerful antidotes comes in the form of vegetables and fruits, as they can help clean up and shuffle out many toxins, but all the steps within this book are critical. I will of course be discussing many tips on improving your diet in the bulk of this book. Additionally, the last quarter of the book will highlight other lifestyle and environmental factors that you can improve for maximal health results and more ideal epigenetic expression.

It's so important to give your body what it needs to function properly. You wouldn't put diesel fuel in a premium unleaded engine. It would break down. And yet so many of us do just that to our own bodies by filling them with poor-quality foods.

You've also likely heard by now that consistently high levels of inflammation are unhealthy for the body. In fact, rampant inflammation is thought to be a primary factor behind heart disease, cancers, and other serious chronic health issues. (There is a strong correlation between excessive inflammation and negative gene expression as well.) The dietary tips within this book are largely anti-inflammatory. They will help you balance out your immune system, too, restoring your body's capacity to do what it is supposed to at an optimal level of performance.

All that being said, **every body is unique. You will discover for yourself which combination of foods and nutrients help your body perform at its best.** There is no "expert" out there who can replace your own innate wisdom when you are tuned into what you really need. When you clean up your diet, your senses and awareness of how your body feels when you eat particular things that either work for or against it will become more astute. You'll be better able to gauge what you most need. These pillars should be a solid starting point, but listen closely for what works best for you. This does not mean what your current taste buds or emotions want, but what your body systems want and need. Their signals are trying to communicate with you all the time, but the SAD diet triggers so many disruptive signals that it's much harder to figure out what is really going on until you give them more priority by cleaning up your health.

Please note: because I'm coping with an autoimmune disease in my gut, I follow a more intensive diet than is outlined here. At the outset, this included an *elimination diet* to figure out what foods were negatively triggering my system. It's a really great diet to work with if you have serious health challenges. Even if you ultimately need to go on a more intensive diet like the *elimination*, these four pillars are a fantastic start and the foundation of most healthy diets. This approach within can work well to prevent and even help combat diseases like heart disease and diabetes. If you are challenged by other trickier conditions, I will include more in-depth resources towards the end that you can dig into for further support, including more details on the elimination diet.

Weight Management: Don't Starve Yourself, Indulge in the Good Stuff!

A magic key: keep your mind and intentions on overall health, not weight.

The first thing I'd like to say on the topic of weight management is related to how you perceive it. Putting too much of your mental emphasis on "weight loss" can be a real trap with potential for frustration and disappointment. If you've done a lot of "binge dieting" in the past, the term "weight loss" can dredge up bad memories. Instead, consider framing for yourself the idea that you are *manifesting full-body health*. Keep your attention on what you want to create rather than on what you want to see go away. Focusing on a positive vision for yourself rather than simply reacting to things you are not happy with can put you in an active frame of mind that leads to greater overall health and ultimately more joy.

Don't get caught in a weight "loss" trap. Instead, keep your attention on how you want your overall health to better serve your whole life. The weight balance will almost surely follow.

Early in your process, you might spend time envisioning the life you want to lead, particularly where your physical health is concerned. Journal about specific goals so that it feels real, tangible. These specifics can include topics relating to your weight, but I encourage you to let it be richer than just that one aspect of health. How do you want to feel, more broadly in your life and in the world? Again, it's important to *create* your life from a positive vision, instead of living out of your perceived deficits.

This is ultimately a journey of self-love, of nourishing your whole being: body, mind, and spirit. Nutritional nourishment is only one piece, but it's a critical one. *Love* your way into it above all else. This is the only moment, right now. You get to be "reborn" into a healthier version of you, if you choose. Get whatever kind of support you need to help make it happen. (See the resources section at the end of the book for ways to get support).

For many people, following the steps within this book will result in weight balancing or weight loss, without much need for counting calories or other "diet" strategies. It will even help stabilize food cravings by giving your body what it needs and rewiring your brain in alignment with the better choices you are making. The more traditional "weight loss" approaches of simple calorie counting and food deprivation are certainly one strategy to lose weight in the short term, but if you aren't changing your overall eating habits toward healthier choices that aren't depriving, weight management will only last so long. You can't restrict calories to a substantial degree forever. Your body needs the fuel and nourishment it needs. What's more, calorie restriction in and of itself is just no fun!

For the long haul, the *quality* of the calories you're eating is more significant than the *number* of calories you allow yourself. When you eat high-quality foods that are nutrient-dense (and delicious), your body is much more nourished and, ultimately, much more satisfied. As you move through time, your body will stabilize and balance, and you'll naturally eat closer to the "amount" of food you really need.

It's a huge issue when you eat lots of highly processed foods that can often be what is called "hyperpalatable." Food companies know exactly what makes their processed foods turn on brain-reward receptors in the brain that make us desire to eat more of a given processed food—making it addictive and overpowering the mechanisms that would normally signal when we have eaten enough. Big food manufacturers combine things like cheap fats, carbohydrates, sweets and salts into food items in ways that would not happen in nature but that can seem tastier and turn on receptors in the brain that make you want to continue to eat them past the point of being satiated. This is a highly manipulative practice that has changed the way we eat and in turn decreased our overall health as a society as well as being a major cause of weight gain. As you read through the pillars within, especially the first one relating to eating whole foods, you'll learn more about why it's so important to train your brain and taste centers to eat whole, natural foods to counteract this phenomenon.

Generally speaking, the idea that you must "starve yourself" to be lean is, for most people, absolutely wrong. Indulging in the foods your body needs (and desires) over the cheap, more hyperpalatable foods that dominate so much of our diets nowadays is the magic key to both vitality and stabilized weight. Of course, it's not really magic. It's basic biochemistry.

Let me give you an example of another factor that relates to all this. Refined carbs and sugars are high in calories, but low in nutritional value. Ultimately, it's believed that you have to eat more of these foods to feel like you have consumed what you need to survive. Your body will keep pinging you with signals that it needs more deep nourishment, which you really can't get from sugar. Quality fat on the other hand, as well as veggies, fruits, and good protein sources, are loaded with layers of nourishment that not only fuel the body but also fine-tune all of the intricate systems at work. They provide more nourishment per calorie and therefore are a much better bang for your calorie buck.

You want and need to eat delicious, but also nutrient-dense foods even when you are snacking. When you get enough of the good stuff, it will feel more fulfilling and enjoyable. If you do try to "starve" yourself, at some point, you'll cave into unhealthy cravings.

It's also important to note that yo-yo dieting also has some huge pitfalls. The constant up and down of weight loss, followed by fat storage when you fall off the wagon, can do real damage to your hormones, your adrenal system, and other parts of your body. We also store all kinds of environmental toxins in our body, often in our fat cells. When we lose weight and fat cells shrink, they can release the toxins into our blood stream, if you do this over and over through fad diets, it can really mess things up. This is why it's critical to eat plenty of vegetables, fiber, get adequate protein, and drink plenty of water, as all of these are essential to help to flush out toxins from the body. You'll learn more about this as you read on. Fad diets also often put your body into starvation mode, which "helps" it store fat more efficiently. When the intense calorie restriction inevitably stops, the fat packs back on and often then some, which can lead to negative effects on your body's glucose and insulin levels. Enough said: it's much better to shift away from fad diets toward a more sustainably healthy lifestyle and let the weight take care of itself in the time it needs. For most of you, following the tips within will take you a long way towards your goals.

The ultimate goal isn't to limit your food choices—it's to expand your options!

I must admit, I eat a LOT of food! While some of it is different than what I used to eat, I have loads of mouthwatering, exciting food possibilities in my life. (You'll learn about a lot of really tasty options as you read.) And yet, as I shared previously, my body proportions and weight have balanced and stabilized to a healthy level. I'm 5'11" and weigh around 155 pounds. I don't have too much excess fat, even around the gut where it's most dangerous. My body systems have stabilized, and my weight doesn't really fluctuate past a few pounds. While I do indulge in negative food choices from time to time, I try not to eat them mindlessly or in crazy amounts (to varying degrees of success). My body and my brain have synced up better, and I'm much more in tune with and responsive to their needs. We are now dancing together much more, with far fewer of the craving and addictive responses from my past. It wasn't just me changing my thinking around the cravings either, that was part of it, but when I shifted my diet, my body and brain biochemically changed and helped solidify the changes.

Finally, for some people, there are deeper underlying causes as to excessive weight gain and weight retention, which may require more in-depth work with a highly trained professional, like a Functional Medicine practitioner. Other approaches may be needed, like an elimination diet to check for food sensitivities that may be messing with your body systems. To learn more about other causes of weight gain, check out Dr. Mark Hyman's free e-book *Beyond Food: Other Causes of Obesity and Damaged Metabolism*. You can download it at www.bit.ly/3eL2kpU Again though, for most, this protocol will help tremendously, and the nutritional elements are good for just about everyone.

Body, Mind, and Spirit: An Intricate Interplay

The human body is a vibrant glory of a vessel. There are so many intricate and finely tuned systems inside of us, working in careful concert to keep us not only functioning, but also ideally thriving. From the tiniest micro-elements like our DNA, cells, mitochondria, and even foreign microbes and bacteria (which outnumber our own cells tenfold!), there are so many components and systems whirling around within our bodies every single second. Most of them perform functions critical to our survival and, hopefully, our flourishing. Whether you believe they are fashioned by the heavens, nature, or something in between or beyond, our bodies really are remarkable creations!

There is a constant and wondrous dance going on between what we allow into our bodies and what it has to offer us in return. Everything we introduce into it—that is, into our body, mind, feelings, and spirit—becomes the raw materials from which it is able to generate. That may seem obvious, but it means everything: our thoughts, our hopes and dreams, our fears, our stressors, our current and past traumas, our intentions and prayers, how we move and exercise our bodies, and of course, the nutrients we invest into it (or don't). All of these factors and more make up and significantly influence our physical being. These elements alchemize deep inside us to generate either a vibrant and healthy flow of energy or a stunted or even diseased flow.

Many more of us nowadays—in the age of the blossoming and deepening field of psychology, and mass culture thought leaders like Oprah, et al.—are starting to better understand the negative impacts that stress and lack of movement and exercise have on our body's functions. Many are also better understanding the benefits of mindfulness, meditation, spiritual and personal growth work, a good therapist, and movement practices like yoga or Tai Chi, just to name a few modalities. Serious spiritual seekers have, of course, been at least partly aware of this mind-body-spirit interplay for millennia, but it's now reaching a more widespread and mainstream cultural recognition.

While we frequently hear the adage, "You are what you eat," most people fail to understand the breadth and depth at which nutrition choices impact us. It's not only physical effects like energy levels, disease, weight, health and so on.

Research is beginning to demonstrate that a nourishing diet, or lack thereof, can have a significant impact on our emotional well-being and mood, sometimes as much as or more than psychological or other external stressors. I briefly mentioned earlier of my own surprise at how much it positively impacted my mood. And yet this awareness hasn't been well explored in our mainstream discourse.

While psychological challenges like anxiety, stress, depression, a pessimistic attitude, unhealthy relationships, a lack of social connection, and trauma have a tremendous impact on emotional well-being, lack of proper nutrition can and does cause significant damage to our mental state. More often than we realize, nutritional imbalances can be the driving force of trouble.

Don't get me wrong. As I shared in my own story of healing, it is vital that we engage in a full range of emotional and physical wellness activities that are imperative to a thriving self. Personal and spiritual growth work have a profound benefit on our emotional well-being that can't be avoided if we want a fully realized life. However, I believe that our lack of focus on nutrition is one of the unsung tenets of an emotionally fulfilled life.

For those of us who do believe in spirit, the body is where the soul meets on this plane of existence. I believe that good nutritional practices can be a profound spiritual act, as I'm literally tuning my body to be in a synchronized rhythm and flow with life. Every bite of food I eat, every choice I make, can put me closer to or further from alignment with my utmost potential and highest self. I want to be connected to that flow of life, not mindlessly adrift from it.

Healing Ourselves, Healing Our Planet

Speaking of the flow of life, we too often ignore our deep connection to the whole of the planet when it comes to our food choices. What we eat not only has an impact on our own health, but the health of the Earth and all its inhabitants. We are intricately interconnected to all the systems of the planet, whether we know it or not (and whether we like it or not).

We evolved with this kind of understanding much more engrained into our whole lives and actions. Most ancient cultures had deep working knowledge of the seasons, stars, wildlife, water systems, food supplies and so much more. For most of our ancestors, connection to nature was a sacred and intimate part of our daily lives.

When it came to food, we either hunted, collected or grew our own. We were more closely aware of the consequences of good or bad actions relating to it. If we improperly harvested or damaged the land, we might not have food the next season. If we overhunted the same would be true.

In modern times, we are largely disconnected from where our food comes. We mostly either get it directly from grocery shelves or have it made for us in restaurants. Too many are causally thoughtless about what goes into growing and tending to our food supply. This is having vast and troubling consequences.

Too much of our food is now produced or processed by big agribusiness, looking to make a profit at unhealthy systemic costs—rather than the more sustainable practices of regenerative agriculture which are farming and grazing methods that help reverse climate change and rebuild our depleting topsoil. We overspray pesticides, overuse chemically-based fertilizers, are depleting essential topsoil 10 times faster than it can be replenished, and treat our animals too often in a cruel and unhealthy manner. Our small family farms and ranches are rapidly vanishing, replaced by giant corporate farming operations that have far less care for long term consequences, but instead are looking to financial bottom line profits.

To be fair and accurate, there are many farmers and ranchers who not only care deeply, they also tend as well as they can to their jobs, lands and animals. I grew up on a farm/ranch in Texas and from my family and neighbors have seen the great care most take.

But even with the best of intentions, it can be hard to overcome obstacles when famers face a behemoth of bad food policy, giant multi-national corporate interests and lobbyists who make it increasingly hard to make sustainable and wholesome choices when the whole engine is geared for mass production at the cheapest cost. We subsidize so many things that are not the most healthy, like grains, which you'll see in Pillar 2 are probably not the best food for us to eat at the scale we are.

So, what can we do? Inside the pillars, we will talk at some depth about the quality of the food we eat—making sure to buy organic and more sustainably grown foods. There are real benefits to your health in doing so. But the sustainable future of our planet also needs us to be aware and engaged in protecting the whole chain.

Each of us can of course make a difference with the choices we make when buying food. Spending our money on organic, locally grown and sustainably harvested and raised foods as much as we can will make a difference. Every dollar we spend is ultimately a vote for the kind of world we want to live in. It is urgent for the future of our planet and our health that we pay more heed to this.

We also need to push for policy changes, so that we can better protect this delicate web of ecological systems that need to be in place to feed ourselves and tend to the larger web of life.

We must also educate ourselves more about how the cycles of life work on planet Earth. Spend more time in nature. Grow some of our own food in home gardens when we can. Being connected to nature has proven to be a very healthy and healing part of life. You can read more on this topic later in the book.

Again, as we tune in and tap in to a greater understanding of how our food is grown and raised, how interconnected and interdependent we are to the whole of the planet, and take responsible actions accordingly, we will not only make ourselves healthier, we will be healing the whole of all creation as well. This is a gift that will last for generations to come.

Time to Get Your Awesome On!

As we now dive into the main sections of the book, I want to give you a quick big picture overview of what we will be exploring.

When it comes to nutrition, there are four key pillars we will explore:

1. **Eat a Whole Foods Diet**
2. **Reduce Refined Sugar and Carbs**
3. **Eat Good Fats, Ditch Bad Fats**
4. **Indulge in a Rainbow of Vegetables (and a Bit of Fruit)**

Each of these pillars are interdependent to one another. It's not that taking actions in only one won't give you benefit, it will. But there are abundant benefits that come from the interplay between them. For instance, a higher healthy fat diet is great for most of us, but not necessarily when in conjunction with a high sugar/refined carb diet.

It is a good idea to try and step into at least some of each pillar as you move forward so that you maximize the time and energy you invest into these changes.

Following the Pillars, I also explore some other topics relating to food that will help you live a more healthy life. Some are just further tips to support the pillars, others are different food categories and topics. They include:

- **More tips on food and nutrition:** protein, salt, and snacking.
- **Good gut health:** the critical importance of healthy digestion and how to improve yours.

- **Cooking power tips:** how to make the best use of time to make delicious foods.
- **Proper hydration:** water is a life force; get plenty to keep your body in proper flow.
- **The psychology of change:** how to find the inner motivation to achieve your goals successfully.

While the bulk of this book does focus on nutrition, it is in no way the only thing that helps you manifest a healthy, fulfilling life. I also lightly explore other lifestyle and environmental factors towards that end. There are many important topics, including:

- **Emotional wellness and stress reduction:** exploring the impacts of stress and emotional challenges, as well as how to better cope and cultivate more calm.
- **Minimizing household and environmental toxins:** the dangers lurking in household chemicals, personal care products, environmental toxins, and how to protect yourself.
- **Sunlight nutrients:** why you need to make sure to get enough light for good health.
- **Movement and exercise:** keep yourself moving to maximize vitality and strength.
- **The healing power of sleep:** cultivating a better sleep rhythm for optimal energy and continual healing.
- **Our collective needs:** building resilient community and working for social change.

Ok, now let's get started!

Foundational Pillar 1:
Eat a Whole-Foods Diet

As we begin with this pillar, I want to reiterate the most important overarching key to vibrant health: **eat a whole-foods diet that is as free of processed foods as possible.**

We did not evolve eating the artificial, chemically laced, hyperpalatable foods that line our grocery store shelves today. For millions of years, we evolved eating a diet based on whole foods, not Cheetos and soda. *Whole foods* here means foods that are as unprocessed as possible. For instance, a salad of mixed greens, blueberries, sunflower seeds, shredded carrots, avocado, radishes, and your favorite protein would be whole foods, while something like a boxed toaster pastry—full of highly milled and processed flour, sugar, and artificial flavor additives—is not.

We are adaptable creatures, but the rapid nutritional pivot we've made in modern times is not sustainable for our health. Highly processed foods are new to our repertoire. These pre-packaged foods you find at many grocery stores are designed to be cheap, have a long shelf life, be hyperpalatable to our taste buds and easy to prepare, but most actually come at a huge cost, as they have a tremendously negative impact on our collective and individual well-being.

What's more, the additives and preservatives within them often work against our health. Skyrocketing disease rates have risen hand in hand with these new eating habits, particularly diabetes, heart disease, cancer, obesity, and autoimmune diseases. Many of the ingredients in these highly processed foods are also known to destroy good gut microbes, sometimes more commonly referred to as *probiotics*, which are important to our health. (On the other hand, whole foods are known to feed and build a healthy gut microbiome.)

As we move into the pillars that follow, you will learn more about the negative consequences many of the ingredients in these processed foods can have, especially when it comes to sugar and bad fats. Many ingredients that fill up processed foods are questionable at best, and known toxins at their worst. Most are devoid of nutrients, and some can even contain elements known as *anti-nutrients*, meaning they actually deplete your body of nutrients or block their absorption.

The multinational corporations behind most of our highly processed foods are masters at maximizing profits. They cram these foods full of preservatives to extend their shelf life, put in cheap and often toxic alternative ingredients to cut costs, and fill them with known addictive ingredients. In fact, these companies spend billions of dollars researching which ingredients will suck you in for more. While they reap financial rewards, we pay the price.

If you could do any one thing to improve your health where nutrition is concerned, it would be to adopt a whole-foods diet as much as possible.

What does that look like? If you have many foods in your house that have more than five ingredients on the label, you should probably toss them out. Especially if there are ingredients you can't pronounce or don't sound like they come from nature, that is often not a good sign. These are not things we evolved to eat. Our body typically does not want or need them. There are of course exceptions, but this is a good rule of thumb to follow.

There are countless questionable additives in processed foods. Here is a list of some of the most concerning and common:

- Monosodium Glutamate (MSG)
- Aspartame
- Artificial Food Coloring (FD&C Blue, Yellow, Red, Green, etc.)
- High-Fructose Corn Syrup
- Artificial Sweeteners
- Carrageenan
- Sodium Benzoate
- Sodium Nitrate/Sodium Nitrite
- Butylated Hydroxyanisole (BHA) and Butylated Hydroxytoluene (BHT)
- Potassium Bromate
- White Sugar, Cane Sugar
- Sodium Chloride (Partial Salt)
- Acesulfame Potassium (Acesulfame K or Ace K)

These are just a few examples to give you an idea. If some of these sound like they come out of a chemistry lab, that's because they do. Some of them come from natural foods, but they are highly processed. Do yourself a big favor and skip them! Their toxicity can add up.

Another good rule of thumb is to put your primary shopping focus on the perimeter of your grocery store. It's the edges that usually have the whole foods, like produce, meats, dairy, and so on. The shelves on the middle aisles are where most of the questionable and largely to be avoided processed foods lurk.

In case my descriptions thus far of what highly "processed foods" are hasn't quite clicked for you, here is a list of examples:

- Refined "white" flours and most fresh or frozen baked goods
- Most snack foods, like packaged chips, cookies, crackers, candies, etc. (the naughty "C's")
- Flavored, sugary sodas
- Packaged pre-cooked lunch meats (particularly those with loads of fillers and preservatives)
- Many frozen pre-prepared meals (there are some reasonable brands—look for natural ingredients)
- Fast food

These are a few examples. Again, be sure to check your label and see for yourself how many or few ingredients there are, if more than five, be cautious and limit your exposure.

Certain canned or packaged foods can actually be fine. For example, tomato sauce that has just a few ingredients (especially in glass jars instead of plastic lined cans which can leach Petro chemicals). There are also some companies out there that are producing pre-made foods, like frozen meals, with much more care than the traditional junk we typically see. In a pinch, there are some options for faster food that is made with better quality ingredients. You'll see in much more detail what kinds of foods are good and not so good as I describe them in detail in the next three pillars.

Some of this may seem overwhelming, especially the list of hard-to-pronounce chemical additives I noted earlier. Don't worry, though. If you keep in mind that we are designed to and have evolved to eat a whole-foods diet, and as you read more about the three pillars that follow, the rest of these pillars will fall into place as they are all whole-foods principles and the foods I discuss within each are all whole foods based.

Pillar 2:
Reduce Sugar and Refined Carbs

I know, I know. This pillar is a big one for some folks. I mean, how can you live without those sweet pastries for dessert, those big slices of bread on your lunchtime sandwich, the pasta with your dinner, candy for an afternoon pick-me-up, your morning bagel, and/or that bowl (or two) of cereal? What about that soda to wash it all down? Or all that sugar in your coffee?! It's almost like starchy foods, refined carbs, and sugar are addictive!

In fact, they are. Very addictive. Sugar is one of the most addictive substances on the planet. It stimulates *dopamine receptors* (also known as "pleasure centers") in the brain, which can make it a real challenge to resist if you are regularly hopped up on it. The good news is that once you shift your eating habits, the cravings for this drug dissipate. Would you believe me if I said you might crave a big, colorful salad just as much? Maybe not yet, but you might someday soon. It happened to me, and frankly, I never would have believed it if I hadn't lived it. As you fill your body with the nutrients it needs, and take a break from the crack, uh—I mean crust—you'll start to feel more fulfilled by healthier but still satisfying and tasty options.

If you're still hung up on my claim that those salad cravings will do the trick, don't worry. There are healthier alternatives to satisfy your sweet tooth and carb cravings that we'll explore as well.

Pace Yourself: For those who eat a relatively high amount of refined carbs and sugar, it might be a smart idea to wean yourself off them more slowly. This is because there are risks associated with going cold turkey, such as withdrawal headaches among other symptoms. Many systems in your body are impacted by these shifts, and it can take a while to adjust. As a result, your body's systems might be negatively affected if you make significant shifts too rapidly. If you have any concern, I recommend reducing your intake by one serving every few days until you get down to your ideal range. Pay attention to what your body is telling you. If significantly discouraging symptoms occur, take it easy and slow. We aren't talking simple cravings here, but tangible reactions in your body. An Example: if you feel your energy levels drop too much, or weight coming off too rapidly.

The goal is to feel better, not worse. If you are feeling worse, set the pace of transition to a slower speed. This is your life and your health, and these dietary tips are designed for the long haul. It's worth taking the time to do it right. You will get there! Always consult your doctor if you have any concerns.

Why High Blood Sugar and Insulin Resistance are Big Trouble

While I don't want to get too technical in this book, I do want to give you a little overview of the health mechanisms behind how nutrition impacts your body. This will give you just enough information about how your body works to understand why these pillars are important.

There are three main **"macronutrients"** that your body uses to make energy, they are:

- Carbohydrates (Sugar)
- Lipids (Fat)
- Protein

Each one is critical and offers different support for the body, but a primary function is to provide the fuel we need to operate. We need a good balance of all three to function properly.

Sugars are considered a type of carbohydrate. That's because, like other carbs, they convert to *glucose* (a form of sugar) in the body, which is then used as energy by body systems. When our glucose levels are too high, as often happens when we consume too many sugars, especially from things like refined carbs (such as white flour) and added sugars, the excess glucose is often stored as body fat.

Diets that are high in the refined carbs that so many of us know and love are a modern phenomenon, a major contrast to what we ate for the millions of years as we *Homo sapiens* were evolving. Refined grains and flours didn't even come into our evolutionary equation until the agricultural revolution around 10,000 BCE, and refined sugars, like cane sugar, even more recently. Our ancestors' diets were nowhere near as heavily weighted towards the amounts of simple carbs that we eat today, which are known to be highly inflammatory in the body. And this is a rapidly growing problem as our sugar consumption alone is about 152 lbs. a year for the average American! That's up from 123 lbs. in 1970, and way up from just two lbs. a year 200 years ago. Whoa...

Since our bodies were not designed for this kind of diet, it has done a number on our health. Many of the modern inflammatory diseases which were discussed previously, which are at epidemic levels now, were largely absent through much of human history. Anthropological evidence shows us that the biggest risks and causes of death in the distant past were usually injury and infectious diseases. The modern diet is certainly not the only factor in our health decline as a species, but it is one of the bigger culprits.

For the last few decades, questionable science has told us that dietary fat was the main culprit behind heart disease and diabetes. What we now know is that some of the biggest culprits are refined sugar and carbs, as well as highly processed foods and bad fats (industrial seed vegetable oils and trans/hydrogenated fats), which we'll discuss later. When our blood sugar levels remain elevated from our modern, highly refined carb and sugar diets—and when we consume too much inflammatory bad fat and not enough good fat—it causes inflammation as well as oxidation. These two processes are believed to be the biggest causes of much modern disease. Research shows that those with the highest intake of sugar double their risk of heart disease, some find even higher numbers.

This inflammatory cascade is also one of the greatest causes of weight gain.

So why did we start feeding our bodies so much of these inflammatory substances that cause metabolic diseases and weight gain? Because they are relatively cheap, easy to mass-produce, and shelf-stable. Big food manufacturers looking for quick and easy profits have literally pushed this stuff upon us for decades and spent hundreds of billions on advertisements and buying shelf space in grocery stores to get us accustomed and addicted. Ok, and of course, because buttery, sugary sticky buns taste pretty amazing! (Okay, you now know another of my old and still occasional guilty pleasures.)

What makes glucose create these complications and how does it cause weight gain?

Glucose-fueled energy works when the carbohydrates from veggies, fruits, grains, as well as refined carbs and sugars, are converted into glucose in your body. While we need to burn some glucose as fuel, leading science is showing that glucose may not be the best primary source of fuel for many people. Certainly not in excess.

Excessive carbohydrates and sugars (including one of the biggest dietary evils, high-fructose corn syrup) converting to glucose in our body can raise blood sugar to unhealthy levels and trigger insulin production—the hormone that helps move glucose energy into your cells—in greater quantities than we'd like to see.

The more often your body has to process high blood sugar in this way, the more likely your cells are to become *insulin resistant*. This in turn makes you need more and more insulin to process excess glucose, which is a big driver of diabetes. And since your insulin can't keep up with processing the glucose it doesn't need, it can trigger your body to store the glucose as fat. This is especially concerning when it's the most dangerous kind, belly fat, which is a strong indicator you are becoming insulin resistant and at risk of prediabetes and/or other metabolic problems.

It is believed this might be one of the key ways your body becomes overrun with fat storage. Hence the weight gain. It's not the only factor, but it's worth being very conscious of as you eat.

Because excess glucose, especially from refined carbs and sugars, aren't as dense a form of nutrition as, say, the healthy fat we get from whole foods, which most of us aren't getting enough of, our bodies can hold onto the bad fat created by excess glucose because it thinks it's not getting the nourishment it needs. This is all somewhat of an oversimplification, but gives you a broad idea.

Generally speaking, healthy amounts of fat are a better source of fuel for your body to burn than too much glucose, as good fats (and proteins) are much more dense in nutrients than simple carbohydrates are. (It's very important to note: healthy fats from food are not the kind created in the liver that eventually become stored fat in the body. That happens through a process called lipogenesis, which is triggered in large part by carbohydrates. See below for more.) When you eat excessive amounts of sugar/refined carbs, you can actually feel hungrier and have to eat more because your body is not getting the nourishment it needs. Also, when your body is primarily running on carb fuel instead of fat, you are more susceptible to energy crashes, as glucose burns off more rapidly. You end up feeling like you need to eat more often to avoid getting "hangry" between meals, which triggers your brain to crave a sugary treat. Calorie for calorie, for most people, it's better to tilt your energy source more heavily in favor of healthy fats. They burn more steadily and keep your energy better balanced throughout the day once you've adapted to burning it as your main source. We'll explore fat in more depth in Pillar 3. And as I will say over and over, every body is unique, and there are nuances we must all figure out for ourselves as to what balance is best for us.

Another useful fact: lipogenesis is the process for how the liver converts things like carbohydrates into fatty acids and triglycerides, and when it runs amok, it is a primary cause of high cholesterol and triglycerides in our blood, not how much good dietary fat we eat. As you might have heard, high triglyceride levels are often considered the most dangerous to the body and heart. Overly high glucose levels can also lower your HDL, which is considered a good cholesterol, while creating dangerous forms of LDL cholesterol. (The impact that high levels of blood cholesterol has on your health is a far more complicated topic than we generally hear about, and there is much scientific debate on this subject. It's more than I will delve into in this book.)

Dr. Susan Blum further explains the problems associated with too much refined sugar and carb intake in her book *The Immune System Recovery Plan*:

"In the medical world, a low-sugar diet is also called a low-glycemic diet, and it is the first pillar to lowering the amount of sugar floating around in your blood. When your blood sugar is high, it causes inflammation and damages your immune system[...] A high-glycemic diet raises your blood sugar rapidly and puts you at risk for diabetes, high blood pressure, and cardiovascular disease. It also makes you feel tired and depressed and is one of the greatest contributors to weight gain.

Most important for our purposes, sugar in the blood stimulates your immune cells to actively release inflammatory molecules that travel throughout your body, causing damage and irritation."

As you cut back on these inflammatory elements and your body starts to balance out, your systems will shift. There is a lot of good emerging data, as well as anecdotal evidence from practitioners working with diabetics, that nutrition and lifestyle shifts like these can actually reverse type 2 diabetes (and for most at least improve it greatly). It sometimes takes support from a good practitioner to get there, but there are current numbers that show as high as seventy percent of some type 2 diabetics can go into full remission, no longer needing insulin, while the rest see significant improvement and less need for insulin shots. Pretty impressive!

Some people actually do better with higher amounts of carbs than others, though rarely to the scale of carbs consumed on the Standard American Diet—particularly since so many of us overdo it with highly refined carbs. Some do better with less fat than others. Balance is always key, and you must pay attention to what your body is telling you. If you find you need more carbs than most, let's say because you are an active athlete or do serious fitness work, you might try to eat more starchy tubers (e.g. sweet potatoes), fruits, legumes, and whole grains that are not heavily refined and without lots of additives or preservatives.

As you can see, our body systems can be quite complicated. The bottom line is that when your digestive system is overrun with junk, it can keep a lot of other body systems from functioning in a way that encourages balance and health. Hopefully you can appreciate how important it is to free yourself from the ill effects of overdoing the sugars.

Feel those snack cravings all day long? If you, like so many of us, feel hungry again soon after eating, this can be a sign of both blood sugar dysregulation (i.e., *hypoglycemia* or low blood sugar) and malnutrition. This happens in particular after eating a refined carb- or sugar-heavy meal. Once one makes the shift towards healthier options, many are surprised that their sense of fullness and satiation is sustained for longer. The body is getting back in balance and getting deeper nourishment that is much longer lasting.

I know some of you may feel you are not yet ready for or capable of eliminating the refined sugars, carbs, white flours, and pastas from your diet, but please know that every bite you can cut out will help. As you begin to move in the right direction, your body will become increasingly accepting of the changes. The cravings for them will ease, and your body will feel better. Your taste buds will also begin to awaken to the delights of a more robust array of flavors and sensations from fresh whole foods.

Be brave and bold as you take this on! Your life and vitality are worth it.

HEALTHY EATING TIPS & CHEATS FOR A LOW CARB, LOW SUGAR DIET

*Please note: you can download a handy "**Printable Cheat Sheet Shopping List"** I created just for readers of this book, with key lists and tips included in my tips sections for each of the four pillars. Just print it out to take with you, or save the .pdf to your smartphone so you always have it. Visit: www.nourishyourselfwhole.com/printable-cheat-sheet*

Cravings can be Tricky

Strong cravings are another reason you might want to pace yourself, if you need to, as you scale back your sugar and carbs. Particularly for those of you who eat large quantities of these foods, they can be quite addictive. When your body and mind are used to you eating big, starchy and carby portions at every meal, it can be an adjustment to cut them back. Know that this will shift. For some, it happens more quickly than for others. I personally took a bit longer to adjust. My regular diet at the time included starchy refined carbs at almost every meal. I ate lots of white rice. Almost all my snacks were starchy; I loved my corn chips! It honestly took me a few months to get to my current level, which includes only a few servings of refined sugars and carbs a week, though I have a starchy vegetable every day (see list of starchy vegetables coming up), sneak in a few brown-rice crackers or cassava chips, and the occasional sweet treat.

Know that your body might put up a fight in the first few days of your transition. You may get cranky, headachy, tired, or have other symptoms. This is fairly normal and should pass soon, especially if you are taking the other Pillars seriously by substituting sugars and carbs with good-quality, satiating foods.

I have worked with folks who felt their best path forward was to go all in right off the bat. However, if the idea of cutting out carbs and sugars all at once feels overwhelming and you already doubt that you can pull it off, just take it step by step.

For instance, if you eat carbs at all three meals, plus corn or potato chips as a snack, and cake or another sweet snack at night, it might be better to start slow since you are already pretty entangled. Can you start by removing one of these items for a week? By week two or three, remove two of these items from your daily routine, and so on. Try it out. Your body will start to balance, with benefits really kicking in once your sugar threshold is low enough to recalibrate your systems and let the cravings fade.

Have Sugar/Carb Alternatives on Hand

Another power tip is to make sure you have sweet treat alternatives on hand to help steer your cravings toward better options. For example, you could make chocolate chip cookies out of almond or cassava flour and sweeten them with one of the better sugar alternatives that will follow in a few pages.

*Take pride in your victories, and **be gentle with yourself when it comes to inevitable missteps**.*

Fruit is Great (in Moderation)

The good news is that fruit isn't really in the same category as refined sugar. Because it comes whole and with fiber and many micronutrients, it will digest differently in the body than refined or added sugars and adds many important nutrients to your diet. It's still high in sugar, though, so it's better for most to keep consumption to a maximum of **1-2 servings per day**.

There are leading edge nutritionists who suggest eating fruit only seasonally. Most of us did not evolve eating loads of sugary fruits year-round (except in tropical climates). We ate it only in season, so some are mindful to eat only seasonally available fruits.

Berries and tart citrus fruits tend to be the lowest in sugar. If you are trying to lose weight or have diabetes or pre-diabetes, keep fruit consumption to a minimum, at least while you are getting your body back into better shape.

There are many healthful aspects to fruit—like vitamins, minerals, phytonutrients, antioxidants, and soluble fiber—but you can get many of the same nutrients from vegetables without as much sugar. Charts are available online that show which fruits are higher and which are lower in sugar. The lower the glycemic index and load, the better for increasing insulin sensitivity, which is what you want.

SELF Nutrition Data website is one of my favorite websites to learn about the nutrition content of various foods, including sugar levels and glycemic load: www. nutritiondata.self.com. You can also google a term like "which fruits are lowest in sugar" and you'll see many charts and lists to glance at.

Also, for those that are very physically active, especially who do not have diabetes or a risk, higher amounts of fruit can be more tolerable and even desirable to help fuel energy.

Bottom line though is that fruit is a healthy and important part of most people's diets. It is always better than refined sugars. Just don't go overboard.

Fruit Juice Should be Avoided

Sorry, but fruit juice is not much better than soda pop when it's stripped from the fibers of whole fruit. If it's a concentrate that's been sitting on a shelf for months, it's especially adept at spiking your blood sugar, while also losing many of the vitamins and nutrients which vanish rapidly after juicing a fruit. If you have a juicer to help you juice fruits and veggies fresh, with all the natural enzymes still intact that help better process the sugars in your body, that can be more beneficial, though don't go overboard. Freshly made smoothies that contain the whole fruit is your best bet in this category, the more vegetables you mix with it the better.

Limit Your Grains

Since grains are carbohydrate heavy, most people should probably limit themselves to one serving of whole grains a day (or for some fewer, I have even less than one serving most days and do well), but again, play around with what you can tolerate and what your body needs for this shift to be sustainable. If you are a tri-athlete or into hardcore fitness, you may need more. It's better to go with whole grains rather than refined (i.e. brown rice instead of white).

Gluten-free grains are best for most people. You've likely heard of gluten by now, but for a refresher, gluten are proteins in wheat and some other grains that often stir up the immune system and inflammation in many people's bodies—even those without celiac disease. I talk a little bit more about the troubles with gluten later in the book, but there is a lot of good information out there to help you learn more about gluten. For now, though, I'd suggest you look for whole grains like quinoa, buckwheat, millet, oats, and wild rice instead of wheat breads and pastas. Various companies even make things like pasta out of these grains, which might be an ok alternative on the occasion when you want to splurge.

If you are trying to lose weight or deal with high blood sugar issues, then limit your grains and starches, too.

Standard refined wheat, white rice, and pasta don't do you many favors.

Starchy vegetables are a good substitute that can help fill the refined carb void. They are important because they help provide insoluble fiber and feed your *microbiome*, which is a fancy word for your good, probiotic gut bugs. Some of the best starchy vegetables are: sweet potatoes, yams, jicama, turnips, beets, yucca (cassava), red-skinned potatoes, parsnips, celery root, plantains, and squash (e.g., butternut, acorn, kabocha, delicata, pumpkin, spaghetti). Traditional russet potatoes are ok too, but try to mix other varieties of potato into your mix as russets can be harder on the digestive system than others.

Beans and legumes can be a healthy addition for some too. While they are starchy and higher in carbohydrates, they're also chock full of fiber which helps slow down the process of their conversion to glucose. For vegans in particular, they are a rather essential source of protein. They are also a decent source of some vitamins and especially minerals as well. One important note though, particularly for those with any kind of gut issues (I can't eat them): beans and legumes can be hard on your system, for a few reasons, but in particular for a substance called lectins, which they are very high in. Lectins are hard on our guts and can block nutrient absorption, especially when eaten in significant amounts. To help reduce lectins, you need to soak beans for at least 24 hours, draining and replacing the water a few times prior to cooking. This leaches out many of the lectins into the water to be drained off. Alternatively, you can pressure cook them in something like an InstantPot, which also neutralizes much of this challenging substance. Doing so can make a modest amount of beans and legumes a healthy part of many people's diets.

Cassava flour makes a great corn chip alternative, but be mindful of the oils used to cook them. (Read on to Pillar 3 for more on the best oils to consume.) Again, to find more good alternatives, you can check out my favorite foods shopping list on my website:

www.nourishyourselfwhole.com/resources

Carb Timing

It's probably better to eat your starchy foods either with lunch or dinner. For most people, breakfast is not the optimal time to eat heavy carbs, *especially* for processed and refined ones. We are all a little insulin-resistant in the morning, so it's not a good time to have that bagel. (Though it never really is.) Most people feel lighter and have higher energy during the day when they keep it clean. So stick with vegetables, fruits, proteins and healthy fats for breakfast and skip the cereal, granola and even oatmeal. However, as always, adjust to what you learn works best for your body.

High-Fructose Corn Syrup is Pretty Much Evil!

Even if you're not religious, trust me on this. That means no soda pop! High-fructose corn syrup is the kind of sugar used in most sodas and to sweeten much of the processed food out there. It's cheaper than cane sugar, but research has shown it to be far more detrimental to our health. It's been closely linked with diabetes, heart disease, and a host of other negative ailments. This should be a strict no. Read your ingredients lists, as it is used in many processed foods. Cane sugar is a better bad cheat than anything with corn syrup. If you want to learn more about why high fructose corn syrup is so bad, you can check out an informative article by Dr. Mark Hyman here: http://bit.ly/2AvBoss.

Think of Refined Sugar like Alcohol

Use it sparingly, like you would an alcoholic beverage. It should be an occasional treat, not a daily staple. Better yet, use alternatives listed in the following pages, which are more stable and less damaging, while also being delightfully sweet.

Speaking of Alcohol...

Beer and wine in particular convert to glucose in your blood pretty rapidly, so be mindful of your consumption. Opt for dryer wines and skip beer as much as possible. Hard liquor is a safer bet in terms of sugar (but still not a health food!). If you are going to make a mixed drink, use bubbly water and lemon, lime, unsweetened pure cranberry juice, or some aromatic bitters to flavor your drink, not soda pop or concentrated juices. You'll come to appreciate the fresh flavors. Be aware that if you get a mixed drink at a bar or restaurant, they almost always use the concentrated juices that are very high in sugar and/or mixers that are sweetened with high fructose corn syrup.

Don't kid yourself, though. Excessive alcohol can be very damaging to the body.

Better Sugar Alternatives

When you have the occasional treat, there are some tasty but still somewhat healthier options to sweeten your food. Three of the best alternatives are **stevia, monk fruit**, and **allulose**.

These options contain no calories and won't spike your blood sugar. Monk fruit and allulose looks like and converts into recipes just like sugar, and have a pleasant, sweet flavor not too dissimilar to refined sugar. Stevia comes now in many brands, and some have much more of an aftertaste than others. Look for a whole-foods source that is pure stevia and isn't overly processed for the best flavor and quality. The jury isn't completely in on how these effect your body, but they are likely much better than real sugars when used in moderation. Again, you can check out my favorite foods shopping list on my website:

www.nourishyourselfwhole.com/resources

Here are some other decent sugar substitutes, though they should still be used very sparingly as they are higher in sugar than the three above:

- Coconut Sugar
- Maple Syrup
- Maple Sugar
- Raw Honey

Artificial Sweeteners are a Huge No-No

There is a lot of evidence showing concern for the impact of sweeteners like Aspartame and saccharine on your health. If your goal is to lose weight, think again. These substances can actually cause weight gain. They set your body up to believe it's going to receive glucose, but when it doesn't get anything, it can make you more receptive to converting calories to fat when other calories do come. They can wreak havoc on your metabolism, and new research is showing that they can even mess up your microbiome, among many other troubling health consequences.

Good Alternatives to Refined Flours

Cassava flour, almond flour, and **coconut flour** are some of the best alternatives to mainstream grains when you want to bake. Cassava and coconut are actually *prebiotic*, which means that they can feed good gut bacteria. They really do taste great. There are many good mixes are out there for pancakes, cookies, cakes, pastries, tortillas, that may even be available in your average grocery store nowadays. For the occasional treat, they are a much better option than most other grains.

For a pasta alternative, you can try spiralized vegetable noodles. I like carrot and zucchini. Sweet potato, butternut squash, and beet noodles are good, too. Baking a plain spaghetti squash makes a fantastic alternative for traditional spaghetti noodles, and I find it enjoyable. There is also a product called shirataki noodles made from a Japanese yam that are tasty and closer to traditional pasta in texture and taste. The brand I'm most familiar with is called Miracle Noodles. Almond flour pastas are also available in some markets, typically in freezer section, and are quite tasty for the occasional treat (Cappellos is the brand I like). You can also try alternatives like quinoa or lentil pasta. Again, with the grain-based alternatives, keep it to a minimum.

Emotional Eating and the Warm Fuzzies of Baking

There are so many emotions and often warm memories tied up with carbs and sweets, such as childhood baking with family or friends. Many people have romantic ideas about baking. There can be emotions tied to baking a cake for a celebration or for when someone is having a hard time. You may have baked cookies for the kids, grandkids, or friends to let them know they are loved or had fun, food-based discussions with friends, even recipe-trading for a favorite baked good.

While I do curtail my refined carbs now, because I'm learning to love and respect myself and my body more, I also share many of these deep, seemingly loving feelings about preparing and eating baked goods. My first foray into cooking was baking. I became quite good at it, and it really did create a warm and fuzzy feeling.

I do not completely restrict this part of my life. While I'm full-on gluten-free and don't do any treats with wheat flour, there are the alternatives, as I listed previously (and will delve into further later on). These aren't as bad as wheat flour, so I use them for the special occasions. It's not that we can't indulge at all, but if we really love ourselves and those closest to us, then it's important to take a deep and realistic look at what our food choices, in this case baked goods, are really doing to us. It's time to stop celebrating treats as a glorified comfort and to start celebrating the true comfort that vibrant health can help foster.

Carbs and sugar cravings in particular can be emotionally based and physically addictive. The cravings can be linked to all kinds of emotional triggers, both good memories and challenging ones.

Rather than keeping that train mindlessly rolling along, tend to your psyche and your spirit! You might consider journaling. Ask questions like, "Is there a hole I am trying to fill with these foods? What deeper nourishment does my soul really want?" They call it comfort food for a reason. What is it in your life that you are not tending to? Is it something like stress, challenging relationships, past wounds and/or trauma from childhood or adulthood? Bring more mindful awareness to what is motivating your eating. Doing so often takes its power away and helps you better make positive shifts.

Get support. Consider a good health coach, join a support group, or even see a therapist. Read further on for more tools and resources to get the support you need in the section of the book entitled: "Emotional Wellness, Stress Reduction and Healing Life's Traumas"

Pillar 3:
Eat Good Fats, Ditch Bad Fats

My generation grew up hearing a major fallacy. We were told that eating fat made you overweight and sick. Meanwhile, we heard little about excessive carbs' role in disease creation and weight gain. The evidence is now clear: good fat is crucial to thriving health. When it comes to food, many of the real triggers for disease and excessive weight trend towards sugar, refined carbs, and bad fats.

Healthy fats provide fuel and energy for the body's proper functioning and can have many additional health benefits. They can:

- Lower your risk of heart disease and stroke.
- Reduce unwanted inflammation and blood pressure.
- Decrease bad LDL cholesterol levels, while increasing good HDL.
- Promote healthy functioning of the brain and nervous system.
- Balance metabolism and help establish healthy weight.
- Are required for the absorption of some critical vitamins, the essential fat-soluble vitamins A, D, E, and K.

What Role Does Dietary Fat Play in the Body?

As I mentioned previously, fat and glucose burn differently in the body. Overall, healthy fat is a more sustainable source of fuel for prolonged energy than glucose. Our body needs nutritional, caloric satiation to function properly. It's important to eat enough good fats so that your body isn't overly stressed and can perform its key functions well.

Despite popular belief, having the right amount of quality fat in your diet actually tends to increase metabolism and leads to proper and sustained weight management and health.

When you combine this information with Pillar 2, cutting back on refined sugar and carbs, your body will start to burn stored body fat and get your natural systems back to an appropriate level of function. (And by the way, the healthy fats you eat in your diet are not the same thing as stored fat in your body. Yes, they have the same name, but that does not equal cause and effect.)

In fact, following these pillars should bring your body closer to a *ketogenic state*, in which your body burns more fat ketones for energy. Some of you may have heard of this concept as it's gotten popularized of late. I won't dig into it in this book because it's pretty wonky, but according to a plethora of research, it can be a healthy state to be in for many of us for a host of good health indicators. (If you want to learn more, Robb Wolf is one of my favorite resources when it comes to information about ketogenic diets. He is easily googleable.)

This whole topic of adding more good fats into the diet can be a tough one for many folks to get their heads around because of all the past demonizing of it. To be clear, even the USDA's own food pyramid was recently, however belatedly, revised to include for more healthy fat after years of irrefutable but largely ignored science singing its praises.

Healthy fats are nutritionally dense. This means that they can feed the body more sustained energy per calorie than refined carbs and sugar. Therefore, you get a much better bang for your buck and are able to satiate your body more than you can with carbs and sugar when in proper balance for your unique body. Generally speaking, you have to eat a lot more carbs and sugar for your body to get the energy it needs to run than you do with fat. This is a particularly important point for those who are trying to manage their weight.

Now, here's my first big caveat. **Highly processed, easily oxidizable, and inflammatory industrial vegetable seed oils, which we've been told for decades are better for us, are actually a big villain.** We're talking canola, soy, corn, safflower, sunflower oil, and other so-called "safe fats." (As you read on I'll explain in more detail why these oils are a problem and provide a comprehensive list.)

On the other hand, good-quality fats are essential to our existence. Here we are talking about olive, coconut, avocado, sustainably sourced palm oil, nuts and seeds, and even some quality animal fats, including egg yolks, butter, whole milkfats (cheese) and ghee. (Yup, I said butter.) These are whole-food-based fats. When not eating a source directly from the whole-food, independent oils should be attained through *expeller-pressed methods*, in which the oil is extracted from the nut or seed in one step, relying on force. Examples of this are eating olive and avocado oil, rather than eating the whole fruit (both have their benefits). Expeller-pressed oils are generally healthy and provide a nourishing food. The industrial vegetable seed oils, though, are typically extracted through chemical processes, often using toxic substances.

As I shared in the first pillar, the best rule of thumb for food in general is that the closest we can get to whole natural foods as possible is best for our health. Since we didn't evolve eating highly processed vegetable oils (they've only been around for the past century), we should avoid them and stick to quality fats that we've been eating to great benefit for millennia.

The good news is, by replacing bad fats with healthier ones, you're not having to cut something succulent out of your diet. Instead, you're simply swapping it with a form of fat that is much healthier and actually tastes better. It's a win-win! And by the way, when you try to, say, lose weight by cutting out too many nutrients or calories than you should, it can actually slow your metabolism if not done properly, having an opposite effect.

My second big caveat is that it's very important to take on this pillar along with Pillar 2! They work in conjunction. You don't want to eat a high-fat diet that is also high in sugar and refined carbs. It's a bad mix that creates the kinds of stored fat in your body, especially in areas like your gut, which is known to be disease-kindling. The notorious "beer gut" is actually a kind of fat that dramatically increases your risk of heart disease. It's a sign of metabolic dysregulation. Again, the good news is that it's not the good fats that are creating this problem when they are eaten properly; it's primarily sugars, along with bad fats, that are the culprit.

While our mainstream understanding of nutrition hasn't caught up to emerging science, it's changing pretty rapidly.

It's important to know that fat "cells" in our body are good, when properly fed and functioning correctly, and play a critical role in our overall health and well-being. They:

- Store energy that fuels our overall functioning;
- Are endocrine cells that produce many important hormones;
- Regulate and help steer *neurotransmitters* (the body's brain messengers);
- Function as a communication platform for the entire body.

You want the fat stores in your body to be of the utmost quality. The industrial seed oils that are often oxidized before you even use them work against your body in many ways. Your body needs stable, nourishing dietary fats, both saturated and unsaturated, to function well. Again, source quality is critical! You are what you eat.

The science of how fats and lipids work in the body is far more complex than what many of you would want to read about in a relatively short book like this, so I'll only touch on some key highlights below.

Types of Fat

It is crucial to learn the difference between the types of dietary fats, as some are healthy and others are not. The primary categories, which I will define below, are MUFAs, PUFAs, saturated fats, and the big baddies: trans and hydrogenated fat.

Monounsaturated Fatty Acids (MUFA)

MUFAs are unsaturated fats that are predominantly good for us and important in our diet for achieving good health. They come from sources like olive oil and nuts. Cultures that consume high levels of MUFA fats, such as those in the Mediterranean region, have some of the lowest levels of heart disease in the world. They are also associated with reduced cholesterol numbers and lowered LDL (the so-called "bad cholesterol" number). Omega-9 fats are MUFAs.

Good sources include:

- olives and olive oil
- avocados
- many nuts and seeds
- some animal products (particularly grass-fed, pasture-raised, or wild).

Polyunsaturated Fatty Acids (PUFA)

There are two main types of PUFA: omega-3 and omega-6 fatty acids. Both are unsaturated and important sources of nutrients. In Western cultures, we typically get far more of the omega-6 variety than we need, often ten to twenty times more than we consume omega-3s. Instead of this eye-popping 20:1 ratio, many researchers and experts believe we should consume more of a 2:1 or 4:1 ratio.

As I shared earlier, one of the big problems with omega-6 PUFAs from industrial seed oils is that they are particularly prone to oxidation and can carry damaging free radicals (we'll talk more about oxidation and free radicals shortly). They have more inflammatory elements, can act as hormone disruptors, and can cause problems with your nervous system. Yikes!

In a June 2008 article for the peer-reviewed journal *Experimental Biology and Medicine,* one of the world's leading researchers on omega-3 fats Dr. Artemis Simopoulos explains that "excessive amounts of omega-6 polyunsaturated fatty acids (PUFA) and a very high omega-6/omega-3 ratio, as is found in today's Western diets, promote the pathogenesis of many diseases, including cardiovascular disease, cancer, and inflammatory and autoimmune diseases, whereas increased levels of omega-3 PUFA (a low omega-6/omega-3 ratio) exert suppressive effects."

Foods <u>fried</u> in industrial seed oils high in omega-6 fatty acids are some of the very worst PUFA offenders. They leave your cells and arteries looking just like the fried foods: battered and crusty. Fried foods disable cells from functioning in the short term, and ultimately destroy healthy cells, which can cause heart attacks and strokes.

<u>Eating foods fried in these oils is one of the very worst things you can do to yourself.</u> It creates both short-term

damage and suffering as well as dire consequences in the long term. (You can fry your own foods in certain healthier oils, though. See below for more details.) While eating food fried in these bad oils is the worst of the worst, eating the industrial seed oils themselves generally does the same thing over time.

Omega-3 PUFAs, on the other hand, are now universally believed to be an important dietary staple. These fats are actually anti-inflammatory, helping to cool down an overrun immune system. They should be a far more prominent part of our daily diet. In addition to those listed above, good sources of omega-3 fatty acids include: fish & seafood, flax, chia, hemp, walnuts, some algae, and some grass-fed or pasture-raised animal fats.

Saturated Fat: Is It as Evil as We've Been Told?

We all need some good-quality saturated fat in our diet. Healthy saturated fats from good sources—like coconut oil, sustainably sourced palm oil, or high-quality meats (particularly pasture-raised, grass-fed and well-treated animals!), and even some butter and ghee—can be important dietary staples. Some people are also surprised to learn that vegetable oils like olive and avocado contain saturated fats. Saturated fats help give our cell membranes their stiffness to properly hold together all of their important contents. They help support our immune system, help our cells communicate better, and are required to make hormones. Another plus is that saturated fats don't oxidize like vegetable oils, so they are very heat-stable.

Still not convinced? Well, some of you may be surprised to learn that up to twenty-five percent of known to be healthy breast milk is saturated fat. Saturated fat is not the evil it's been made out to be when well-sourced and eaten according to your body's needs.

When consumed in conjunction with a diet low in refined carbs and sugars, high in vegetable fiber, and high in good MUFAs and PUFAs, saturated fats can actually reduce inflammation in the body. As part of a well-balanced healthy diet, and not overdone, they are critical nutrients.

The amount of saturated fat we need can shift from person to person. Again, everyone is unique. A very small percentage of people have a gene that could make saturated fat less beneficial when consumed in excess and can cause some of the cholesterol issues I mentioned earlier. If you are worried, talk to your primary care provider—or better yet, a good Functional Medicine doctor, who can perform genetic tests to see if you are one of the few that might have an issue. We all need some saturated fat in our diet, but if you're concerned, you can keep tabs on how you feel consuming different amounts, you can monitor your good and bad cholesterol, and if you're really concerned, you can keep your primary focus on fats like fish, olives, avocado, nuts, and seeds and you should still get enough saturated fats.

The Big Baddies: Trans and Hydrogenated Fat

The type of fat that is now universally understood to be toxic and linked directly to coronary artery disease is called trans fat, or hydrogenated fat. Trans fats and hydrogenated or even partially hydrogenated oils are highly processed foods, typically made from industrial vegetable seed oils. They are processed in a way that allows them to be more "shelf stable" and thus cheaper and easier to produce and store for long periods of time to maximize food company and grocery store profits. These fats should be avoided at all times. Be mindful, even when your nutrition label says "0 trans fats," the food can still include some, as the FDA allows for 0.5 grams or under to be listed as "0." The more processed foods you eat with these bad oils, the more the grams will add up, and any amount will do damage. With this in mind, it is better to read your labels for bad oils listed as ingredients than to do a quick scan of the nutrition facts.

The lesson here: ditch the margarine and bring back the butter! (Just don't go overboard with it.)

Dangers of Bad Fat: Oxidation

A key risk of consuming bad fats occurs because of a process called oxidation. Oxidation is a disaster for the body, and another main driver of diseases, including heart disorders, cancer, and strokes. This is one reason that most vegetable oils are a problem. The bad ones oxidize easily.

Oxidation is damage caused by oxygen. It's like when apples or bananas turn brown from air exposure. This happens with fats, too, and it's essentially what happens inside your body when you eat oxidized oils. It's kind of like rusting on the inside. The ensuing *oxidative stress* creates *free radicals,* molecules that are inflammatory and can damage your body. Most of the bad and highly refined industrial seed vegetable oils mentioned cause great risk of this happening inside you (excessive carbs and sugars also contribute to this cascade).

Heat is a particularly robust enemy for these low-quality vegetable oils, as it can cause them to oxidize even further. Unfortunately, they are often exposed to heat both in their initial processing and through cooking. It's a double whammy that keeps amplifying the trouble. Oxidation can be an issue with some healthy fats as well, but we will talk about how best to cook with and store them for best results later in the tips section.

Another downside to bad fats and oxidation relates to brain health. At least sixty percent of your brain is made up of fat. *Essential fatty acids* work to help the flow and communication for all the little firing synapses and neurons inside. This is important to know, as low-quality vegetable oils provide a poor substitute for quality fats and can attack the brain in multiple sectors. Regular consumption of low-quality vegetable oils can lead to an all-out assault on your brain, which is also the organ in our body that is most susceptible to oxidative stress. You want to fill up your brain with good-quality fats that provide for the best "current" possible. Turns out you think the way you eat, too!

You might be surprised to hear that around the turn of the twentieth century, most of these highly refined vegetable seed oils didn't even exist. As manufacturers discovered a method of taking oil out of traditionally non-oily plants, they became cheap to produce and therefore became the predominant forms of fat in most people's diet (once again, profitability can often trump health). There was also a lot of bad science put out (often funded by the same industries that profited from the sales) and a big-money marketing and lobbying push (by those same industries) to prop these low-quality oils up on their false altar. And here we are today, with junk filling up most of our processed foods and used far too frequently in our cooking. Hand in hand with that, metabolic disease rates have been skyrocketing since we switched to using these kinds of fats.

Cholesterol: Some are concerned about fat as a cause of high "bad" cholesterol. As I mentioned in Pillar 2, cholesterol that makes its way into your blood is primarily made in the liver. You might be surprised to learn that the dietary cholesterol contained in the food we eat does not have much impact on the cholesterol in our blood. These two substances that share the same name work very differently in the body. What's more, the kind of saturated fats that end up in our blood and arteries come mostly from carbs and sugar (and sometimes from excessive protein), not so much from fat. It is also converted in the liver and sent into our blood supply.

As I previously mentioned, I am on a very high-fat diet and have seen my cholesterol numbers get even better as I switched to good sources of this macronutrient. This is true for most people, but stay mindful of the caveats I mentioned.

Learn More About Fat: For those interested, you can really geek out on the various types of fat our body needs, and those it doesn't. There are so many roles fat plays in our thriving health. If you are interested in learning more, I'd suggest reading the work of Dr. Mark Hyman and Dr. Catherine Shanahan. Google their names along with the word "fat" for a myriad of informative articles and videos. Here are a couple of good ones to get you started:

- "Dr. Mark Hyman on Eating Fat to Get Healthy – with Lewis Howes" (YouTube video): www.bit.ly/2Ouit53
- "Dr. Cate Shanahan – 'Practical Lipid Management for LCHF Patients'" (YouTube video): www.bit.ly/2OuiOER (This one's really only for those who want to geek out on the deep science. It's in depth but fascinating.)

HEALTHY EATING TIPS AND CHEATS FOR A DIET THAT INCLUDES GOOD FAT

*Please note: you can download a handy "**Printable Cheat Sheet Shopping List**" I created just for readers of this book, with key lists and tips included in my tips sections for each of the four pillars. Just print it out to take with you, or save the .pdf to your smartphone so you always have it. Visit: www.nourishyourselfwhole.com/printable-cheat-sheet*

Best Types of Fats and Oils to Use

- Olive Oil (always extra virgin, cold-pressed)
- Avocado Oil
- Coconut Oil (virgin)
- Tallow and Lard (from good sources, like grass-fed animals)
- Butter and Ghee (Clarified Butter) (grass-fed is best)
- Palm Oil (sustainably sourced)
- Smaller amounts of cold- or expeller-pressed, unrefined nut and seed oils, such as macadamia, walnut, and sesame. Flax, chia, and hemp are also considered to be decent sources.
- Full-Fat Dairy. For those that can tolerate dairy, this can be a good source. (Organic, grass-fed sources are best.)
- Quality, Grass-Fed and Grass-Finished or Pasture-Raised Animal Fats.

Diversity is important, so mix it up and get a variety each day.

Fats and Oils to Avoid

- Canola
- Soy
- Corn
- Sunflower
- Safflower
- Cottonseed
- Grapeseed
- Sesame (unless used cold-pressed in things like salad dressing, but not in processed foods or to cook with)
- Margarine (even if it says "olive oil" read label and note they usually contain other less than ideal oils too.)
- Most non-stick cooking sprays (some new companies are using avocado or coconut oils, which may be better)
- Anything labeled "Vegetable Oil," "Shortening," or with words "Hydrogenated" or "Trans Fat" on label.

Remember, almost all processed foods contain one form or another of these toxic fats.

How Much Fat to Eat?

Many functional nutrition experts say anywhere from 30 to 60 percent of your caloric intake should come from healthy fats. After all, you must replace the simple carbs you cut out in Pillar 2 with something else. As with everything, your body is unique, and what will give you the energy you need is also unique. Play around with amounts as you lower your sugar and carb intake to see what you need to feel energized. I've found that I hover around 90-130 grams of dietary fat per day. An example of this: olive oil contains about 14 grams of fat per tablespoon.

Cooking Temperatures for Fats

When cooking with oils, you want to keep them below their smoke point. When they get past their smoke point, they start to form dangerous free radicals, which I discussed earlier when I talked about oxidation and will share even more in Pillar 4 on vegetables and fruits. Avocado oil is one of the best for cooking at higher temperatures. Quality tallow and lard can also be good. Peanut oil can be good for frying, but be careful to get a high-quality source as peanuts can be full of mold and *mycotoxins*, toxins produced by fungi. See the chart below for a handy smoke point reference guide. However, please note that I have seen various contradicting smoke point levels for assorted fats, so just be safe and don't cook very often at high heats.

Fat Smoke Points:
Avocado Oil 520°F
Ghee 485°F
Palm Oil 450°F
Coconut Oil (expeller pressed, refined) 450°F
Coconut Oil (extra virgin) 350°F

Macadamia Nut Oil 390° F
Beef Tallow 400°F
Duck Fat 375°F
Lard 370°F
Olive Oil (extra virgin) 320° F
Butter 350°F

Much of this data is from: John Barron, "Healthiest Cooking Oil Comparison Chart with Smoke Points and Omega-3 Fatty Acid Ratios." Baseline of Health Foundation. http://bit.ly/2DakQYT

Meat Quality Matters

As Dr. Mark Hyman says, "We are what we eat... and what our food eats." If you are not a vegan or vegetarian, then be as mindful as possible to eat good-quality animal products. Pasture-raised meat is often more than ten times higher in beneficial omega-3 fatty acids than traditional grain-fed or grain-finished varieties are. Most of our cattle, for example, are grain-fed for at least the last six months of their life. This doesn't make their beef inherently bad. In fact the protein from all relatively clean meat is beneficial to our bodies. But if we are supposed to avoid grain, why wouldn't we think it would impact us when our animals eat it? As often as possible, go with the best quality and try out the grass-fed varieties when you are able and go for leaner cuts of grain fed animals. Be careful though as they often label meat as grass-fed when they actually feed the animals grains for at least a few months at the end of their lives. So make sure to check for "grass-finished."

There are certain cuts—like traditionally considered tougher pieces, such as chuck roast, brisket, chateaubriand, oxtail, etc.—that are naturally higher in omega-3s even in grain-fed livestock, so those can be better cuts to choose when you are eating grain-fed beef, especially if you eat the fat. You can also go for leaner cuts when eating grain fed.

Raw Nuts and Seeds

Raw nuts and seeds can be a great source of fat and other nutrients. I want to emphasize the word "raw," though, because the fats within them can easily turn rancid and/or oxidize, especially when heated too much. At the very least, if you eat roasted nuts, make sure they are dry roasted. Many companies roast their nuts in bad industrial vegetable oils, which can cause double the trouble. Some research has shown health benefits even with roasted nuts, so just do the best you can and still make them a part of your diet.

Be mindful, and don't overdo the nuts. A handful a day is generally more than enough as we don't need too much of the special types of fat they contain. While very important, these fats can be overutilized and cause some trouble.

Many people are not aware that it's important to store nuts in the fridge. They will last longer this way and better protect the delicate oil from going rancid.

One final bonus step for nut super-eaters. With some nuts, like almonds, it's a good to soak them for a day before eating. Purchasing raw, unpasteurized nuts will allow them to slightly sprout as well when soaked, which makes them even more nutritionally beneficial. Problematic, anti-nutrient chemicals that are not good for our digestive system in excess, like phytic acid and some lectins, will leach out into the water prior to eating. Twenty-four hours is usually enough time. Add in a tablespoon of apple cider vinegar to the water when soaking and it can also help cut down on any possible fungal growth. If you like your nuts on the crunchier side, you can always dehydrate them after soaking.

You can perform an internet search to learn much more about the benefits and how-to's of nut and seed soaking and sprouting.

Olive Oil

It's very important that you always buy extra virgin and cold pressed olive oil. When the oil is of a lower quality, the heat and chemicals used during processing damage the oil. Store your oil in a cool, dry place away from sun or heat, and try to buy it in a bottle that is darker in color, which helps protect it from oxidizing and going rancid. You also want to cook with it using low to medium heat as it doesn't have as high a "smoke point" and can oxidize in the pan (there is competing data about the smoke point, with some researchers and experts saying it actually has a higher smoke point, meaning you can cook at higher temperatures.) Shelf life for a good quality olive oil after opening is not as long as some, you want to use it up within a few months after opening.

Olive oils are great for salad dressings, for light sautéing, and for drizzling on your favorite foods and snacks. Whole olives are of course also a healthy food. One of my favorite snacks is to make some fresh olive tapenade and use it as a dip or to add to foods and sauces.

It's important to note that olive oil is unfortunately one of the most counterfeited oils in the world. It's not cheap, so many companies lie and either blend it with other cheaper oils, like canola, or fake it altogether. And restaurants often say they use olive oil, but it is also a blend. Be mindful that you are buying yours from a good source. You want to know how old the olives are and that you aren't getting a mishmash of various fruit form various times and places. You may or may not see a date, but check the label to make sure it has just one country of origin, not multiple. If it doesn't say, the odds are higher that it's not as good. And beware, "bottled in" is not the same as "grown in" so don't be fooled. In this case, and many others, you do tend to get what you pay for. A good quality oil is key for health so this is an area I invest in.

Power tip: If you have the $$ to invest in premium olive oil that gives you the detailed nutritional content and sourcing of the oil, it's worth it. You can typically only find these kinds of oil details in specialty oil stores (there aren't a lot of them) or at online retailers. They will reveal details like country of origin, oleic acid content (higher the better), polyphenols or biophenols (higher the better), free fatty acid (FFA) content (lower better, keep under .4%), Peroxide value (lower better, keep below 12), and more. My favorite is a local store that also sells online called Amphora Oils: www.amphoranueva.com (they also have blow-your-mind-good flavored balsamic vinegars).

Avocado Oil

It is the mildest in flavor of the cooking oils and can withstand some of the highest cooking temperatures. Avocado oil tastes good and is great for light frying or roasting if you want to occasionally fry something at home. It's also great for sautéing and for salad dressings. I like to toss my potatoes in a little of the oil and roast them in the oven.

Note that even if you have sensitivities to avocados, you might have an easier time with the oil as it's only one component of the whole fruit, and many have issues with the flesh rather than the fat. It's worth trying out unless you have an allergy.

Coconut and Palm Fats

For coconut oil, you generally want to get a virgin product, which may not be stated on the jar. One way to tell if coconut oil is virgin is to check for "solid" oil instead of a "liquid." That said, the oil will only remain solid up to 76 degrees Fahrenheit, so, depending on where you buy it or what time of year it is, the oil may look liquid on your store shelves. If this is confusing, you can try the oils from the following brands: Artisana, Nutiva, and Dr. Bronner's, all of which are of good quality and can be found at most health food stores and many regular grocery chains.

I typically use coconut oil either as a dip (stir in a little sea salt and use it with veggies or the occasional rice cracker) or to stir-fry with veggies or eggs or dishes that could use a light tropical flavor.

Another good source of fat is coconut milk. It has a delightfully rich and creamy flavor. It's a cooking staple in many cultures; Indian and Thai foods are two prominent examples. I love it in smoothies and soups. Coconut milk also works well as a creamy element in salad dressings, which is one of my favorite uses for it. You can also find coconut cream in stores, which is a fantastic alternative to whipping cream.

Medium-chain triglyceride oil (or MCT oil as it's more commonly listed) is another very nutritious oil that is a component of coconut oil. This boosts energy, improves brain and memory function, and suppresses appetite. You can buy the standalone version of this oil, which means the MCTs are extracted from the coconut oil and made into straight MCT oil. While it's not really designed for cooking, you can put MCT oil in smoothies, coffee, salad dressings, or just eat it by the spoon. Again, look for virgin varieties.

Sustainably sourced palm oil is another good, vegetable-based saturated fat that has a high smoke point. The flavor is very nutty, and it might be an acquired taste for some. A good brand is Nutiva. Their palm oil is made from a protected farming forest, as compared to many other palm oil producers who cut down and destroy rainforests, habitat and other pristine places to source their product.

Butter and Ghee

It's always best to get grass-fed butter or ghee. Kerrygold is a good-quality, grass-fed brand you can find in many markets. A good butter or ghee is more yellow in color than white. In addition to the quality fats they provide, butter and ghee are a great source of vitamin A, a crucial fat-soluble vitamin that's hard to get from many modern foods. It also has many other fat-soluble vitamins and trace minerals and contains MCTs. When grass-fed, butter can contain high levels of a cancer-fighting compound called *conjugated linoleic acid.*

For those of you not familiar with ghee, it's a form of butter that's slowly heated and separated from the water and milk proteins, making pure oil. It's milder in flavor than butter and, in my opinion, has a smoother texture. It's very nice and doesn't contain any of the milk protein *casein,* which can cause food sensitivity even for those who don't know they have it. Ghee contains two to three times more vitamin K2 than butter, which is another important nutrient that is hard to get elsewhere in the diet. It's also very shelf stable since there isn't any water in it. It has a relatively high smoke point so you can sauté with it.

I make a dip from ghee and Himalayan sea salt for carrots, celery, jicama, and other fun veggies. It's a delicious, filling, and energizing snack.

Good-Quality Fish

If you aren't vegan or vegetarian, wild-caught fish or certified, sustainably farmed fish are your best sources of beneficial omega-3 fatty acids. Stick primarily to smaller fish, like salmon, anchovies, sardines, and trout. Larger fish, like tuna and swordfish, tend to be much higher in mercury and other pollutants, as they continually eat smaller fish that have accumulated their own mercury and toxins, which then amplify as they are stored inside the larger fishes' bodies. This can really add up as our oceans have become more and more polluted.

Please note, though, that omega-3s are fragile! I never cook fish at temperatures over 340 degrees Fahrenheit. That is the point at which the omega-3 oils will begin to oxidize. I find that baking at 340 degrees cooks it just as well as higher temperatures, though you'll need to add a bit more cook time. If you cook your fish on the stovetop or grill, use medium to medium-low heat. Low and slow is key.

Vegan and Vegetarian Omega-3 Options

For vegans and vegetarians, avocado, olives, coconut oil and milk, nuts and seeds, flax, chia, and hemp are all great sources of fat. Try algae for one of the most well-rounded sources of omega-3s. Chia, flax, and hemp do have some omega-3s, but they aren't very bioavailable (meaning the ability to absorb well into your body) and aren't the ideal forms, though these foods still can be good for you for other reasons.

Full-Fat Dairy

When I was younger, skim milk was all the rage. It rolled in as part of the low-fat craze discussed previously. Now that we know quality fat is an important part of a healthy diet, dairy can be a good addition for many. It's actually the fat that contains most of the healthy parts of dairy. Many of the fatty acids found in dairy are actually protective against disease. Again, though, many people are intolerant of the milk protein found in dairy called casein. Some are lactose intolerant, which is a sugar found in milk. Therefore butter and ghee can be good alternatives if you suspect a sensitivity. Both are largely free of these two substances.

If you decide to go with dairy products, make sure to get them hormone- and antibiotic-free. Purchase organic and grass-fed products as much as you can. Larger animals treated with hormones and antibiotics live longer and accumulate more toxins as they age, which can and does leach out into the milk and then into your body when you ingest it.

80/20 RULE:

I first heard this phrase from Chris Kresser, though many in the Functional Medicine world are aligned with and use the idea. The thrust is, you spend about eighty percent of your time eating to your highest chosen standards. The other twenty percent of the time, just do your best, even allowing for some fun.

So, if you are on vacation and eating out or with

---

friends is too complicated to maintain every element of your lifestyle shift, relax a little.

If there are easy, healthy choices on the menu, of course choose them. Don't sweat it too hard, but pick the things that sound like the most fun. For example, why waste your twenty percent on bad fats in a salad dressing when those fats don't even taste good? Ask for olive oil and balsamic vinegar.

The body is resilient and amazing. It can and does handle quite a lot of negative input. The more you cut it a break and feed it what it needs to thrive, the more you will reap benefits and the more it can handle the occasional curveballs thrown its way. But when it's time to have fun and options are limited, don't sweat it!

Tips for Restaurants

Ask for steamed vegetables, and then get a side of butter or olive oil to add to it yourself, rather than the cheap and toxic industrial vegetable seed oils they typically use to sauté. Many good restaurants will also swap out the vegetable oil for butter or olive oil when sautéing if you ask. (*Hint:* tell the server you are a good tipper ahead of time so they aren't as annoyed by lots of questions and special requests. Yes, I'm that guy!)

Another thing that I sometimes do when I think there might not be good options for fat at a restaurant is to bring my own olive oil and vinegar. I like to eat well when I go out, and while many restaurants now have olive oil, I don't want to risk not having yummy food if they don't. Instead, I sometimes bring very small two- to three-ounce glass jars with lids, filled with my favorite oils and vinegar. Then I have something to pour on my salads, over steamed veggies, and so on.

Fried Foods are Toxic!

This bears repeating. **Generally speaking, eating deep-fried foods at restaurants is one of the worst things you can do to your body.** Not only do restaurants almost always use bad oils for frying, they are using them for days at a time. Most restaurants don't change their oil more than once a week (that is all that is required by law). These oils become rancid quickly and get more and more oxidized by the day, amplifying the badness. Chances are good you are giving yourself a boatload of toxins that overwhelms your body as it tries to process and clean it up (typically unsuccessfully). The negative results are immediate and have long-term consequences. Skip it!

There are some fats that do a better job of frying, but most restaurants generally don't use them. In the fairly distant past, most frying was done using tallow or lard, which are actually more stable and therefore not as unhealthy as industrial seed oils. When I was a kid, I remember loving French fries from McDonald's. They were fried in tallow, which tasted much better as well. Then the anti-saturated fat fad set in and turned the whole industry around, likely to our great detriment.

At home you can fry by using fats like high-quality, grass-fed lard or tallow or, at lower temperatures, coconut or avocado oils. Even peanut oil holds up better, but again, you have to find a good clean source of it.

Fast Food Fats

Do I really need to write this paragraph after all we've been through together? Don't do it! Fast food restaurants are of course cutting every corner possible to bring you the cheapest (i.e., most profitable) food and the worst of the worst quality. Their burgers and fries are full of refined carbs, sugars, terrible fats and oils, and mostly low quality meats, all to bring you the perfect storm of body-destroying anti-nutrition.

Just skip it and get an awesome, colorful, nutrient-dense salad. If you need something fast, find a big salad, even at a fast food joint, as many now carry them. When I do eat at fast food restaurants, I choose places like Chipotle, where I can choose what I want off the line and only get the healthier items.

Storing Fats and Oils

Keep your liquid unsaturated oils in dark containers in dark, cool, and dry places away from the stove. Heat, sunlight, and air can increase their oxidization and even cause them to become rancid. Try not to buy more than a few months' supply of oil to keep it fresh and try to use it within a month or two after opening. That's when it will be the most fresh. Some specialty oils might need to be kept longer as they are occasionally used. Don't sweat it too much, but you can extend an oil's shelf life by using special air-pump caps made for wine bottles to pump out the air after each use. These can be found on Amazon or at most wine shops.

Always Read Your Labels

Many processed foods, even salad dressings, use poor-quality oils to save a buck. Be mindful that this adds up in the body, so you should avoid as much as you can. Read your labels to find alternatives for salad dressing, there are a few brands like Primal Kitchen and Bragg that make versions with good oil.

Pillar 4:

Indulge in a Rainbow of Vegetables (and a Bit of Fruit)

Ah, veggies and fruit, the nutrient powerhouses! The more vegetables we can eat, and fruits to a lesser degree, the better.

In modern life we are faced with far too many toxins and irritants and not enough nutrients to help counteract them all. However, fresh vegetables and fruits are chock-full of nourishment called *micronutrients*, which include vitamins, minerals, antioxidants, and phytonutrients. They also provide quality fiber and some wholesome carbohydrates for energy. These nutrients provide critical support for the body's vast array of working systems deep down at the cellular level. They help:

- convert food into energy,
- repair cellular damage,
- heal wounds,
- strengthen bones,
- clean up damage done by bad fats, sugar, and a whole host of environmental toxins,
- support a functioning immune system, among many other crucial supports for our body's needs.

More than a third of our population—some studies show over half—are deficient in basic vitamins and minerals. This is according to Recommended Dietary Allowance (RDA) standards, which are relatively minimal requirements based on population averages rather than populations that are more healthy. There are health experts who believe that some of the RDA standards are simply meant to keep us out of acute disease states rather than ideal health. Considering the amount of nutrients we actually need to thrive, not just survive, most of us are woefully undernourished in these important micronutrients, especially given our toxic modern world.

Vitamins, Minerals, Antioxidants, and Phytonutrients as Disease Inhibitors

Taking vitamin and mineral supplements can have some benefit, but they are not often adequate for the deep nutrition our bodies need. These supplements are often poorly absorbed and not highly bioavailable, meaning that a rather small proportion of the micronutrients activate and enter the bloodstream. No single or even multi-nutrient pill can contain the thousands of micronutrients that are available from a whole food source. These many micronutrients carefully and powerfully interact with one another, dancing around the body, performing many interrelated acts of support for us.

With this in mind, vegetables can be indulged in liberally (aim for 6-10 servings per day with a wide variety). Fruit intake needs to be a bit more carefully monitored. As I mentioned earlier, most of us with ancestors from temperate zones didn't evolve eating fruits year-round. We ate them in season. Most fruits are higher in sugar, and there can be problems with that. Thankfully, whole fruit typically comes with a lot of fiber that helps slow down sugar absorption, which can help moderate blood sugar spikes more so than refined table sugar. Due to the many vital nutrients within them, fruit should certainly be a healthy part of most people's diets, but be mindful of how much and how often you eat them. A handful or two of lower-sugar berries is more than enough for a day of good nutrition and sugar balance. One or two servings of fruit a day are plenty for most people unless you are more physically active. If you are challenged with blood sugar issues like diabetes, you should be particularly careful. And if weight management is an issue, you should be mindful as well.

Keep starchy vegetables to a minimum as well, especially if you are more sedentary, as they have a greater capacity to break down into sugar than other vegetables. These include vegetables like potatoes, corn, and beans. One or two servings a day is best for most here, too unless you are very physically active.

Antioxidants and Phytonutrients

In addition to vitamins and minerals, which you've likely heard about in some capacity since grade school, vegetables and fruits contain important micronutrients like antioxidants.

These substances literally put out fires in the body. That's their job. They help undo at least some of the detrimental circumstances and choices we inevitably face in our lives, whether they are food choices, environmental exposures, stress, or other less than ideal factors.

Phytonutrients refer broadly to compounds that only come from plants. These are often protective substances that the plants create and use to shield themselves from the assorted harms they face. It's thought that various plant species contain over 100,000 different kinds of phytonutrients. In fact, they form the basis from which more than forty percent of all our medications are built.

Many of these phytonutrients work to protect and nourish us. They are critical to our health. While they are lesser known in terms of mainstream awareness, some of the more commonly understood phytonutrients include carotenoids, ellagic acid, flavonoids, resveratrol, glucosinolates, and phytoestrogens.

For example, there are more than 600 carotenoids that generate the yellow, orange, and red colors in fruits and vegetables. These carotenoids produce not only color, but also a variety of very specific nutrients we need. That is why it's important to mix it up when it comes to your vegetable consumption! **Get in a wide diversity of colors every day**. The rainbow isn't just for beauty on your plate. It is also the key to nutritional diversity. There is no pill, supplement or single, isolated substance that can match the important spectrum that comes from various whole vegetables and fruits.

How Free Radicals Do Their Damage and How Vegetables and Fruits Can Help Clean Them Up

Free radicals are unstable atoms that form in the body in relation to oxidation. A little exposure can actually be good to build up your body's internal strength, but too much causes a lot of trouble. When there are too many, free radicals can be extremely reactive and destructive to the body's proper functioning. As I shared earlier in the book, our genes aren't set in stone, they are highly susceptible to environmental factors like these. At the cellular level, free radicals can do serious damage to DNA, cell membranes, lipids, carbohydrates, and protein molecules. When the ratio of free radicals to antioxidants gets too high, along with other factors that help regulate them, oxidative stress can really get us into trouble. As we discussed earlier, this oxidative stress is one of the main drivers of diseases and a whole host of challenges in the body.

Some of the free radicals contributing to oxidative stress form from normal metabolic processes in the body. Even exercise can cause them to form. Some cooking processes can add to free radical production, like grilling meat. The blackened parts of grilled meats are chock-full of free radicals. In addition to the food-based free radicals discussed in Pillar 3 relating to bad fats, we can get added exposure to them from environmental toxins, chemicals, water pollutants, radiation (like X-rays and air travel), cigarette smoke, pesticides, air pollution, and a whole host of other toxins. We are all exposed to these on a daily basis, to varying degrees. Obviously, the more exposure you have, the more at risk you are of developing excessive free radicals along with their negative effects. It is of course important to minimize your exposure to these dangerous influences, but here is some good news. **Antioxidants are the primary method of wrangling and neutralizing free radicals, thereby helping to shift oxidative stress**.

Antioxidant molecules can safely interact with free radicals and terminate the chain reaction that causes oxidation before other fundamental and healthy molecules are damaged in the body. As such, they are essentially one of the body's primary antidotes to disease-causing forces. And what is a primary source of antioxidants for our bodies? Yep, as I shared earlier, vegetables and fruit.

Since we know vegetables and fruit are full of antioxidants, then it goes to figure that the more vegetables and fruit we eat, the more hard work they can do to clean up free-radical damage in the body. If we get enough— depending on the toxic load, of course—antioxidants can stop damage before it even starts. This is why, in our modern life with so many toxic exposures, it's so important that we eat as many vegetables (and some fruit) as we can.

Antioxidant supplements may be a different story. The jury is not yet out on the pros and cons of high-level supplemental antioxidants.

Fiber: Vegetables and Fruits Contain Some of the Best Kinds

Another great benefit of vegetables and fruits is the important fiber content. Fiber can help bulk up the stool, including detoxified "bad stuff" our body needs to flush out, and move everything through the intestines more efficiently. It also helps minimize blood sugar spikes by slowing sugar breakdown and absorption, it helps feed good gut bacteria that provide numerous benefits for our healthy functioning, and more.

There are two types of dietary fiber, both of which are important to the body: soluble and insoluble fiber. Great sources of soluble and insoluble fiber include:

- leafy, green vegetables;
- yams and sweet potatoes;
- carrots and other root vegetables;
- squash;
- fruits with an edible peel, like apples and pears;
- berries;
- seeds;
- nuts.

Most of the scientific research linking high fiber to good health has studied diets high in veggies and fruit. Conversely, the fiber that is added to processed foods so marketers can slap a "high in fiber" on the packaging, can be detrimental to our health. We hear a lot about the fiber in grains, but the jury is still out there as well. Research has shown grain fiber to have anti-nutrient effects by blocking vitamin and mineral absorption. Your safest bet is to get your fiber primarily from vegetables and fruits, along with some nuts, seeds, and legumes.

Weight Loss and Detox

Vegetables and modest amounts of fruit are also an important part of weight management. You can eat large servings of vegetables without taking in too much calorically. They also help keep your body systems flowing and maintain your metabolism as part of a healthy whole-foods diet.

You may have also heard the phrase "detox," relating to good health. This is a term that encapsulates many different functions in your body that help clean up and flush out toxins. The nutrients in vegetables and fruit are critical supports for your body's detox systems, especially to help the all important detox organ, the liver. As the nutrients within vegetables and fruit (and quality protein) travel around your body, they help boost our natural systems and ultimately clean up a whole host of bad actors.

The fiber in these foods then help capture and flush out the cleaned-up toxins.

As a result, vegetables and fruit (and drinking plenty of water) are literally the most important things you can add into your diet to help you detox better. (Of course we also want to work hard to avoid chemical and toxin exposures so there is less to clean up.)

For these and many more reasons, robust consumption of vegetables and some fruit are a cornerstone of any healthy diet. Dive in! Experiment! Learn what you love and go from there.

HEALTHY EATING TIPS AND CHEATS FOR A DIET RICH IN VEGETABLES AND FRUIT

*Please note: you can download a handy "**Printable Cheat Sheet Shopping List**" I created just for readers of this book, with key lists and tips included in my tips sections for each of the four pillars. Just print it out to take with you, or save the .pdf to your smartphone so you always have it. Visit: www.nourishyourselfwhole.com/printable-cheat-sheet*

Cooking and Preparation

Generally speaking, it's best to steam, not boil, your veggies. Boiling can leach a fair amount of vitamins and nutrients into the boiled water so that the resulting vegetables aren't as nutritionally dense.

You can also sauté them, though try to do so at lower heat and with good fats or liquids. I've found that steaming many vegetables, followed by a very quick sauté (in the same pan, just dump the water), makes for a very tasty dish. I typically drizzle some avocado, olive, or coconut oil over mine before sautéing. If I'm feeling a little wild and crazy, I might even use butter or ghee!

If you need your salt, add a good-quality, whole sea salt just before you plate your food. If you add it too early while cooking, the salt will pull the moisture out of your veggies and make them cook in their own liquids, which can make them more mushy and less tasty, especially when sautéing.

Some veggies bake especially well, like tubers and root vegetables (ex. potatoes, parsnips, carrots, radishes, etc.).

You can roast many other vegetables in the oven, too. I love to lightly toss things like broccoli, green beans, brussels sprouts, zucchini, and bell peppers with good oils and roast them in the oven. (Keep the heat below the smoke points mentioned in Pillar 3 so you won't damage the oils.)

Raw vs. Cooked

Some health practitioners recommend that most of the vegetables we consume be raw. Others say vegetables in any form—aside from perhaps smothered in liquid processed cheese—are good for us and that we should mix it up. Who is right? Well, raw vegetables and fruit have more of their nutrients and enzymes still intact. Though cooking will damage or release some nutrients, it can also make them easier to digest and therefore the nutrients more bioavailable. Variety is fine, so try to mix it up.

For some people who can't handle raw vegetables, perhaps due to a digestive challenge, cooking vegetables is the only way to go. If you use the preparation tips provided earlier, you'll still get plenty of nutrients. You may even find that with this diet, over time you can rebuild your capacity to handle more raw veggies. That is what happened to me.

A fun fact: the key nutrients in some fruits and veggies actually increase when cooked. For instance, tomatoes actually gain more of the beneficial *lycopene* antioxidant when cooked. There's a great book that goes into detail on how best to prepare and store your fruits and vegetables for maximal nutrition. It's called *Eating on the Wild Side: The*

Missing Link to Optimum Health by Jo Robinson. She also has many good tips on her website: www.EatWild.com.

Fresh, Frozen, or Canned?

Generally speaking, if you live somewhere that you can get fresh produce that wasn't picked and shipped too long before the purchase date, like a farmer's market with local produce or a grocery store that carries quality produce, this will by far be your best choice in terms of taste and nutrients.

There are certain circumstances in which flash-frozen vegetables and fruits (in your grocery store's freezer aisle) can retain as much as or, in some cases, more nutrients than fresh. Broccoli is a good example, as some of its most beneficial nutrients degrade just a couple of days after harvesting. This is especially true if you live somewhere that vegetables are not very fresh. You can typically tell by how healthy they look on the shelves—if wilted, withered, or turning "off" colors, they are not very fresh.

"Fresh" veggies and fruit are often picked before they are ripe and shipped great distances, allowing for degradation in taste and nutritional value. Frozen vegetables and fruit are often picked at peak ripeness, and flash-frozen very soon after picking. Frozen doesn't work for every occasion or recipe, but consider it a viable option. One note: try to eat frozen vegetables within the first three months after purchase as their nutritional value can still degrade over time in the freezer.

Canned vegetables, however, should generally be skipped. They lose a lot of nutrients in the canning process and are often filled with unhealthy preservatives and toxins that leach from the plastic lining in the cans. Exceptions include tomatoes, pumpkin puree, some beans and legumes, but be sure to avoid cans that are not free of bisphenol A (BPA), as the acid in the tomatoes can increase that toxin-leaching process. Glass jars are a much better option. I talk about this further in the section "Minimizing Environmental Toxins" later in the book.

Going Organic

As much as you possibly can, buy organic. The pesticides, herbicides, and fertilizers that are used to help produce conventionally grown crops are shown to be particularly toxic to humans. These chemicals can mess with hormones as well as increase your risk of cancer, diabetes, and a host of other issues. Meanwhile, there are some solid studies that show organic vegetables have higher levels of many nutrients, including antioxidants.

I realize it's not always possible to buy organic, especially depending on where you live. The Environmental Working Group (EWG) has done a great job of identifying the biggest "problem" fruits and vegetables on their annual "Dirty Dozen" list. They do rigorous testing and research to identify the most pesticide-ridden fruits and vegetables, the ones we should buy organic, every year.

Here is the recent Dirty Dozen list, with the worst culprits first:

- Strawberries
- Spinach
- Nectarines
- Apples
- Grapes
- Peaches
- Cherries
- Pears
- Tomatoes
- Celery
- Potatoes
- Sweet Bell Peppers
- [Dis]honorable Mention: Hot Peppers.

Please note, this list can change a bit from year to year (though it tends to stay pretty consistent). Check www.ewg.org for the most recent list.

Try to get organic varieties of these for sure, or adjust recipes and swap items on this list out for cleaner alternatives. If you can't find fresh organic versions of these foods and you really need one of these items, consider looking for organic frozen.

Speaking of cleaner conventionally grown options, EWG also has a list called the "Clean Fifteen," listing the least contaminated. This year's includes:

- Avocados
- Sweet Corn
- Pineapples

- Cabbage
- Onions
- Sweet Peas (frozen)
- Papayas
- Asparagus
- Mangos
- Eggplant
- Honeydew Melon
- Kiwi
- Cantaloupe
- Cauliflower
- Broccoli

On a related note, EWG makes a great set of smartphone apps for identifying more and less toxic foods in general. You can also check out their food score website at www.ewg.org/foodscores. Here, they rank the health of food items you might find at the grocery store.

Fermented Veggies and Fruits

By this point I'm sure you've heard about the benefits of probiotics. There is plenty of research that shows that eating probiotic-rich foods can likely help most of us improve the health of our guts, or our "microbiome." This in turn boosts the entire body, including the immune system. Even with some of the best probiotics in pill form, you aren't going to get anywhere near as many of the good bacteria as you can with something like traditionally fermented sauerkraut, which can have trillions of good bacteria compared to mere billions in pill form.

You can make your own fermented vegetables fairly easily. You can Google how-to videos. If this feels daunting, you can buy them premade in many health food stores. There are sauerkrauts, but also fermented pickles, carrots, and a whole host of veggies and even fruit, like shredded apple, that you can enjoy. Be aware, though, that we are not talking about the "pickled" sauerkraut or pickles on the shelves in the middle of the store. They are devoid of probiotics. Instead, the probiotic forms are kept in the refrigerated sections and should say something like "probiotic food" on the label. It is an acquired taste for some, but worth the effort. These are very nutrient-dense foods, and your gut will love you for it.

Start slow with probiotic foods. If your body isn't used to probiotics, it can be a tricky adjustment. Start with a teaspoon daily, and if you do well, increase from there. Eventually, you might enjoy a half a cup of fermented vegetables per day. There is a small percentage of people (myself included), who just don't do well with probiotics for reasons we won't get into here. This is not because probiotics are necessarily bad for our individual bodies, but because they can cause intestinal discomfort for people with underlying gut issues. If you find that even a slow introduction doesn't settle well in your gut, you may have to skip the fermented vegetables.

Prebiotics

Speaking of probiotics and the microbiome, one of the best ways to build it up to a healthy status is to feed your existing gut bugs what are called *prebiotic foods*. These are types of food that are especially beneficial when it comes to cultivating a healthy microbiome. They especially thrive on these kinds of foods. Research has shown that feeding your gut bugs these prebiotics is an even better way to build up a healthy microbiome than taking probiotics. Some of the foods highest in prebiotics are:

- onions,
- Jerusalem artichokes,
- starchy tubers like jicama and cassava (yucca),
- dandelion greens,
- raw garlic
- leeks.

If you can tolerate them, eat prebiotics as often as you can.

Herbs and Spices

Be liberal with herbs and spices in your cooking. They are some of the most nutrient-dense foods we have, and there is a wide variety out there to try. Fresh herbs generally have more nutrients, but dried ones are still a good choice. I tend to enjoy herbs and use a heavier dose than most recipes call for. If it says two teaspoons of oregano, I double or sometimes triple it. I enjoy the strong flavors and appreciate the health benefits that come along with it.

You can mix it up, too. Try out different herbs or spices with different foods and see how they taste. I like to use the smell test. (I may have made this up, or it could actually be a thing. Either way, it works for me.) This means that I smell the base food, then the herb or spice, and if I like the combo, I try it out. This is my own method, and it's completely unscientific! More often than not, though, it works out beautifully.

Salads

As you read this pillar, you may be wondering how you're going to enjoy vegetables liberally, as I suggested. Salads are a fantastic way to eat lots of veggies (and fruit), for a real powerhouse of a nutrient-dense meal. They are great for lunch or dinner, even at work. You can easily make your own ahead of time and bring it with you. One smart trick for hyper busy folks is to prepare an entire work week's worth of salads ahead of time in air-tight containers, like large glass mason jars. Google "mason jar salads" for some really fun ideas.

To your salads, mix in a variety of different types of lettuce, even some darker greens or red leaves varieties like radicchio. I usually add in additional veggies like radishes, carrots, cucumber, cabbage, celery, fennel, fresh turmeric, leftover cooked veggies, nuts, seeds, avocado, sprouts (which are super nutrient dense), roasted and cooled cubed butternut squash, blueberries, leftover salmon, garbanzo beans, or another protein, maybe even a little grain like quinoa. There are so many combinations to try. My salads are hearty and robust!

I typically make my own salad dressing, as most of the dressings in stores contain the bad oils we talked about previously in Pillar 3. To do this, I shake together some apple cider or balsamic vinegar, and/or lemon juice, and add salt, pepper, a pinch of herbs, and then mix it with oils like olive, avocado, cold-pressed sesame, walnut or macadamia nut. Another fun option is to use coconut milk, which is one of my favorite fat bases; it makes for a creamier dressing. Making my own salad dressing takes about two minutes, tastes great, and I know it's good stuff. I use one part base flavor (i.e., vinegar and/or tart citrus) and two to three parts oil. Again, the fats are what make it most satiating. If you want to get really fancy, try mixing it in a blender and adding in fun elements like strawberries or avocado. This makes your dressing thick, creamy, and super tasty!

If you're short on time, there are some companies like Bragg, Primal Kitchen and Chosen Foods who make quality dressings with one of the good fats, avocado or olive oil. Be aware, though: even dressings that say "olive oil" on the front label, which is of course also a good fat, often use a blend with canola or some other less preferred option, so as always, read your ingredient labels.

For the most nutrient-dense types of lettuce, look for varieties with open leaves, which generally have much higher amounts of phytonutrients. Closed-headed varieties have fewer, though cabbage and the radicchio/chicory families are two exceptions. Red, purple, and reddish-brown leaves have the most phytonutrients, followed by darker greens. The lightest green generally have the least (iceberg lettuce has almost no nutritional value, it's not unhealthy, but skip it). Also, the more intense the flavor, then likely greater is the lettuce's nutritional value.

Another power tip: If you dress your raw greens a bit before you eat the salad with a little olive oil or the dressing, waiting up to ten minutes, the oils will help bring out both flavor and nutrition, making the nutrients even more bioavailable.

Smoothies

Another great way to get a lot of vegetable and fruit nutrition is from smoothies. If you recall from Pillar 2, we are all a bit insulin-resistant in the mornings. Instead of reaching for a breakfast laden in refined carbs and sugars, consider the fiber and micronutrients of a smoothie. It really is a great way to start your day and kick it off with loads of nutrients for your body.

Green smoothies that are made up of seventy percent or more of vegetables are what you want to aim for. If you have a good strong blender, you can process standard items like cucumber, kale or other dark leafy greens, fats like coconut milk or avocado, yogurt, some blueberries, lemon, and maybe chia seeds or nuts, along with a little ice. Frozen fruits and vegetables can work great. One of my favorite items to add in is zucchini, which to me adds a really silky texture and taste. There are countless recipes and smoothie cookbooks online. Look for "paleo smoothie recipes" to find the healthiest.

Sweet Potatoes vs. Russet Potatoes

Just because you're leaving the Standard American Diet behind doesn't mean you can't enjoy the occasional russet potato (though russets tend to have more anti-nutrients that can block vitamin and mineral absorption in your gut). However, consider that, despite their name, sweet potatoes have a lower glycemic "sugar" load than russet potatoes, by up to fifty percent. They also have more phytonutrients and double the antioxidants. Those with the darkest orange flesh have the most nutrients and are often called "jewel yams" in grocery stores. Baking, roasting, or steaming sweet potatoes can double their existing antioxidants, but boiling reduces this. (Steam instead if you want mashed sweet potatoes.) Other good potatoes options are red potatoes and colorful varieties, like purple potatoes.

Garlic

Garlic is a powerhouse of antioxidants, particularly the antioxidant *allicin*. **Cut, chop, or crush the garlic clove and let it sit for ten minutes before cooking with it.** This helps release an enzyme that protects the good stuff from being destroyed by heat and helps you realize the best nutrients. If you don't wait, heat will kill some of its beneficial nutrients.

Be Adventurous, Mix It Up!

Bottom line: try new veggies and fruits. Keep the colors flowing. If at first you don't like something, give it a chance. Your taste buds will often adjust. Especially as you cut back on sugar, both your taste buds and your brain will start to recalibrate. The subtle flavors that you might not have noticed or the robust one you might not have tolerated before will start to shift.

Four Pillars Wrap-up: A New Lease on Life Awaits!

These Pillars will take your health a long way forward. There is so much research to back this information up, but ultimately, your body will tell you what is working for you. Play around with your implementation of the four pillars and pay attention to how you feel. (Remember, there might be an adjustment period where you feel weird, with symptoms like cravings and withdrawal headaches, but give changes time to settle in.)

In making these changes, you should start to feel more vibrant and fulfilled, and you should start to notice results fairly quickly. This is good news, because when your body works well, it's a whole new world.

I know there was a lot of nutritional information to read within this book. For some, it may feel daunting to take all this on. Remember, though, that every small step you take should improve your health. Taking it all on step by step is a smart idea. In fact, research suggests that this is the way long-standing habits are formed. You don't have to push through all at once. Even baby steps will make a difference! And thankfully, your body will start to feel better and that will be its own motivating reward.

Be gentle with yourself as you engage with this new eating approach. It's far too easy for many of us to beat ourselves up when we don't meet goals or slip up or get confused, but that is human nature. Change can take time. Keep the negative self-talk down. Celebrate even the little victories and accomplishments and set yourself up for an ultimate victory by making self-love and wellbeing your bottom line.

This is your life, you deserve to treat yourself well. Do so, and you'll see life blossom. Your whole world will start to treat you well, too.

Nourish Your Self Whole

Additional Healthy Eating Tips

The four core pillars are by no means the only factors that contribute to optimal health. While they do appear to have the biggest bang for the buck where nutrition is concerned, there are a whole range of steps we need to take to keep our bodies, minds, and even spirit in top shape. Implementing the four core pillars will likely make significant improvements to your health. I would suggest starting there and really homing in on the tips and practices laid out. As you are inspired and able, the additional tips that follow can be woven into your daily choices to improve your life and vitality even further.

In this section of the book we will explore:

- **More tips on food and nutrition:** protein, salt, and snacking.
- **Good gut health:** the critical importance of healthy digestion and how to improve yours.
- **Cooking power tips:** how to make the best use of time to make delicious foods.
- **Proper hydration:** water is a life force; get plenty to keep your body in proper flow.
- **The psychology of change:** how to find the inner motivation to achieve your goals successfully.

Again, as with the first section of the book, the information here isn't exhaustive. I'm trying not to overwhelm you with data. I include enough information to hopefully give you the fundamentals for success and in some cases resources to dig deeper if you'd like to learn more.

Protein

Like our other two macronutrients, fat and carbohydrates, protein is an essential part of a healthy diet. Your body uses it to build and repair tissue, hormones, enzymes, and many other crucial body chemicals and processes. It can help you manage your weight, lower blood sugar, support detox, and keep muscle mass in good balance—among many other benefits. In fact, your organs, muscles, and tissues are largely made up of protein. It is essential to almost every function in the body.

So, it makes sense that we need to constantly replenish our body's stores of good-quality protein. However, just because a food source says it contains protein doesn't mean it is a complete or optimal protein source. There are twenty one different primary *amino acids*, the building blocks of protein, which are all critical to our health. Some protein sources have better varieties of amino acids than others. Your body can actually produce some amino acids, but it cannot make nine of them, which means you must get those from your diet, and in necessary proportions.

Each amino acid performs different functions in the body, so we want and need a well-rounded variety. Meat offers the most comprehensive array of amino acids. It's good to mix up sources, though, especially if you are vegan or vegetarian. Vegans and vegetarians must be vigilant and careful to get a well-rounded set of amino acids and combine sources properly. Kris Carr and Ocean Robbins are good educators and writers on how to eat healthily as a vegan.

Amino acids in protein are important for detoxing as well. To put it simply, detox is the way your body takes things that are toxic, and removes them from your body. Critical pathways of your body's detoxification systems require these nutrients to function properly. They are an especially critical element of an important detox phase that supports your liver in shuffling toxins out of your body.

Good sources of protein:
- Grass-fed, pasture-raised, or wild meats. Any meat will give you good protein, however opt for grass-fed and grass finished or pasture raised when you can. You may have to ask if the meats are grass finished as they can list "grass-fed" on the label, but that is only for part of the animals life, they often "finish" with months of grain and the label can be misleading. (*Power tip:* organ meats like liver and kidney are some of the healthiest foods you can eat for a variety of nutrients. They are far more nutritious than the muscle meat we typically eat nowadays.)
- Fish
- Eggs
- Yogurt or Kefir
- Nuts and Seeds (especially almonds)
- Beans and Legumes (non-GMO, organic soy can be good for vegans and vegetarians who can tolerate it)
- Cheese (goat cheese is one of the more tolerable varieties)
- Bone Broth

- Grass-Fed or Pasture Raised Animal or Vegetarian Protein Powders

How Much Protein to Eat?

This is a question that isn't completely settled, even in the nutrition and forward-thinking Functional Medicine communities. Generally speaking, between 20 and 35 percent of your caloric intake is thought to be a good range for protein consumption. This could be between 50 and 90 grams a day for the average person. If you undertake vigorous physical activity, then you need more protein than sedentary, elderly, or chronically ill folks.

For perspective, a can of tuna contains about 25 grams of protein. An 8-ounce steak has about 56 grams. One cup of black beans is about 15 grams. One large egg is about 7 grams. Half a cup of almonds or a serving of quinoa offer about 15 grams. As you can see, if you eat meat, it doesn't take as much as many people think to get your daily needs.

Most experts agree that you should spread protein throughout your meals and that you don't want to go overboard on protein. There is some good research that suggests that if you have too much protein at one given meal (over 40 grams), it can cause your blood sugar to spike, among other health detriments. Experiment with your body and see how much protein you need in comparison to the other two macronutrients, fat and glucose. Regardless of how to look at it, it's a critical part of a healthy diet.

Is Salt Really the Enemy?

Salt is one of the most demonized nutrients around, but in fact, whole, natural salts are critical to our health in a variety of ways and should be a part of a balanced diet.

Whole salt helps keep us hydrated and wards off dehydration. It offers important trace minerals and helps balance electrolytes. It also helps key muscles and organs function properly, including a properly functioning digestive system, which is critical for nutrient absorption. We must replenish our bodies' salt stores as we lose much of it through urination and sweat.

It's very important to note, though, that most of the "table salt" a typical household uses, and certainly most of what is added into processed foods, is only a portion of whole salt. It's a highly processed version that is heated to over 1,000 degrees and stripped of most of its complex trace minerals and other nutrients. It is then bleached before being bottled up and labeled as salt. What's mostly left is the split element, sodium chloride, and some anti-caking agents that are usually not desirable for consumption. It's important to note that most processed foods use these types of cheap salt.

These processed salts are a cause for concern, and in part may be responsible for many of the negative health consequences we've heard about for decades. For example, some research has shown this stripped-down version to be more of a factor in raising blood pressure than whole salts would be.

Whole salts, particularly whole sea salts, offer an array of complex nutrients. They also taste quite nice.

Some of the best types of sea salt are:

- Celtic Sea Salt
- Himalayan Sea Salt
- Real Salt (which contains the natural, good nutrient iodine)

Some argue that eating sea salt from our increasingly contaminated oceans could pose a risk, as they may carry some of those pollutants. If you are concerned, you can try the Himalayan sea salt and/or Real Salt brand as both are mined from ancient sea beds that are largely devoid of modern ocean contamination. Celtic brand sea salt claims to only gather salts from more pristine northern waters. These are the only three brands I've researched, but that doesn't mean there aren't plenty of other good brands out there.

Whole sea salts are an important part of a healthy diet, but of course, don't overdo it. Although note that if you take on this whole foods diet, you won't be getting nearly as much salt as the average person, as most of the salt (the bad kind at that) in the typical persons diet comes from the highly processed foods most people consume. So especially if you are eating a whole foods diet it can be important to make sure you add in enough good salt to keep a healthy balance. Many in the leading-edge nutrition and medicine communities feel that between 1.5 and 3.5 teaspoons of sea salt per day is a healthy amount, depending on your lifestyle and personalized needs. For instance, people who exercise and sweat heavily will deplete more of their natural salts and have a greater need to replenish.

For more thoughts and research on salt, including ideas on how much is the right amount, Chris Kresser has some thoughtful articles at http://bit.ly/2K49mYj.

Also, leading cardiovascular researcher, Dr. DiNicolantonio, has written a well-researched book called *The Salt Fix*, with loads of in-depth analysis that might surprise you. Check it out at www.thesaltfix.com.

Snacking

For many of us, especially in the industrialized West, snacking feels like a birthright and is a deeply engrained part of our lives. Far too many of us graze throughout the day (and often way too late at night). Some of this is psychosomatic, while some of it can come from a real biochemical urge.

Biochemically, many feel the need to snack so frequently because of blood sugar crashes that come when they are on a higher-glucose diet, as described in Pillar 2. This causes your body to send out hormonal signals to eat and replenish the glucose coffers when they are running low, which happens far more frequently when you are indulging in too much glucose overall in your diet. Some people with blood sugar regulation issues cannot keep from snacking.

As you integrate the four main pillars into your life, your cravings and your blood sugar crashes will become less common and/or less intense. For most people, it is actually a good idea to let at least four hours pass between any kind of eating. This allows your small intestines to determine that it's safe to release food particles into the colon, which helps keep up a healthy flow of digestion and good gut "motility." Snacking can trigger your digestion to slow as the body senses more coming in. As a result, it holds on to what's currently in your small intestines for a longer period than is desirable.

Snacking is also a cause of weight gain, as it doesn't allow your digestive system to fire off the hormones that signal your body to burn fat rather than new food. This is an oversimplification, but when your body gets the signal that you are taking in more food, it keeps trying to store that excess energy as body fat. So, you want to give your body time to burn off excess glucose energy and begin to burn fat. If you are constantly snacking, it's not able to do so as effectively.

A few tips for when you feel like you will need a snack. First, try to bring healthy snacks with you, especially when you are travelling. If you like heartier snacks, try things like carrots (or some other veggie) with hummus or olive tapenade. Both dips are hearty and filling. Find alternatives that include some fat or even a little protein, which can satiate without sending your blood sugar back up as much. I bring little ghee packets with me, and maybe a can or pouch of wild salmon.

If you are feeling hunger pangs but want to avoid snacking, a great "biohack" is to go for a short walk. This can help reset the craving. Again, though, once you change your diet for the better, these cravings should taper at least some as a result.

Leaving Space Between your Meals

As I just mentioned, we didn't evolve eating around the clock like many do now. Many nutritional researchers now believe it is important to leave windows of time between eating. I mentioned previously regarding the spacing between meals to allow at least four hours between meals for proper digestion. There is also good research about fasting longer. While some people do very fancy fasting protocols, going 24 hours or more without eating on occasion (which has been shown to extend lifespan and health in some good research), it is more broadly believed that we should allow at least 12 hours between meals at least once every day.

For most that happens at night after your dinner and before breakfast. But some people stagger their meals by eating only breakfast and lunch, or like me, only lunch and dinner. I like to aim for a 14 to 16 hour window. Again, there is research that shows this can be very valuable to health, including blood sugar regulation and mitochondrial function. There are people with blood sugar and other health issues for whom an extended period may not be beneficial. Again, always talk to your healthcare provider. But the 12 hour window is probably safe and desirable for most people.

Good Gut Health: *How to improve your digestive system, deal with food intolerances, and other food related health conditions.*

In an ideal world, we'd be able to eat any and all "healthy foods" with no worries. Unfortunately, that isn't the case for many of us. Food intolerances and allergies are rampant. These intolerances cause our immune system to kick into high gear, which can lead to all kinds of troubling consequences. This all happens in large part due to poor gut health.

Good gut health is one of the most important influences to our overall health. The gut is where we process and absorb all of our nutrients. When its microbiome is not in good shape, it can be the driver of disease and a whole host of bodily ailments. By "gut," I'm referring to our stomach, small intestine, and large intestine—the main players in the human digestive system. Modern medical science is increasingly understanding that our small and large intestines are the home base for our immune system, too. It's currently believed that about eighty percent of the immune system is housed there.

What you allow into your body, especially your mouth, has a great impact on gut health. Many foods, including sugar and bad fats, can do great damage to your intestinal lining. This not only keeps you from absorbing nutrients as you should, but it also fires up your immune system in ways you don't want it to, creating systemic inflammation. Researchers in the field now better understand how all this works.

When too many internal and external stressors are introduced into your body, it can often wreck your gut. One of the biggest problems that comes out of this is a well-researched condition called *intestinal permeability* or "leaky gut," as it's more popularly known. This condition causes the "spaces" in your gut wall, which are normally a tight junction that allow nutrients to pass into your body from digested foods, to open up too wide. This in turn allows in food particles that either shouldn't be entering altogether or particles that are too large. Your immune system then targets these suspect particles, some of which might otherwise be healthy actors, tagging them as bad actors and creating an inflammatory immune response to try and wrangle the assaulting foods out of your body. Generally speaking, this is one of the main ways your immune system works to keep you healthy when anything it doesn't like comes in, like a virus or the free radicals we talked about earlier.

You can probably imagine that, over time, having your immune system constantly engaged from intestinal permeability would be a problem. This constant inflammatory assault actually does more damage to your already dysfunctional intestinal lining and your whole body in a variety of ways.

I've described the problems with over-rampant inflammation earlier in the book, so I won't go too much further into the details on all this, but it isn't good to be in this state. Leaky gut negatively affects far too many of us. When it remains entrenched for a long period of time, your whole body can start to degrade. As I said earlier in the book, many think it's just bad genetics causing these problems, but very often, the root cause can be related to poor gut health.

You might think that since you don't feel many symptoms directly in your gut, you are fine, but in fact, a whole host of symptoms throughout the body, as well as major diseases, like auto-immune and many others, are now believed to be tied to a dysfunctional gut. Examples include joint pain, skin conditions, allergies, thyroid problems, arthritis, nerve pain, headaches and migraines to name a few. The good news is that when you clean up the gut, it can calm the waters significantly. Many other health challenges you might be experiencing can subside or even disappear.

The Microbiome and Probiotics

Another key driver of good gut health is a well-balanced *microbiota* in our large and small intestines. Our microbiota, or "gut bugs," are both related to the popularly known probiotics. These gut bugs number in the trillions and include good and bad bacteria, yeast, viruses, and other tiny organisms. We evolved with these critters and couldn't survive well without them. Microbiota have been found to be crucial to our immunologic, hormonal, and metabolic balance. They even help regulate our emotions! Current research into the microbiome shows some remarkable new discoveries. According to Chris Kresser:

The gut-brain-microbiome axis connects the body's central nervous system (CNS), which houses the brain and spinal cord, with the enteric nervous system (ENS) of the gastrointestinal tract. This axis facilitates bidirectional neural, hormonal, and immunological communication between the gut and brain. The microbiome is the third key component of this axis. It serves as an intermediary between the gut and brain, since the microbes it contains produce metabolites that relay messages to both organs.

— From "Is IBS a Gut-Brain-Microbiome Axis Disorder?" The Kresser Institute

It's a whole new frontier in health and medicine. We are learning how important it is to keep our microbiome strong. Antibiotics are one of its biggest enemies. Even one round can kill off much of our bacteria, and it can take months or even years to recover (if it even can without some guided help). Many other factors can positively or negatively influence it, including sleep, environmental toxins, poor diet, and stress. While all of these factors need to be looked at and addressed, making sure we feed the gut bugs well is important.

One of the main ways we can feed our microbiome well is through gut-bug-friendly foods called prebiotics (outlined in Pillar 4). As a reminder, good sources of prebiotics come from foods with lots of soluble and insoluble fiber, like onions, garlic, chicory, Jerusalem artichokes, leeks, and dandelion greens. Search Google for whole lists of additional good prebiotic foods. Fermented foods are also helpful as they contain pro- and prebiotics to help train your gut system.

A Cure for Gut Problems: The Elimination Diet

Some people who are in the throes of major diseases or body challenges, particularly those suffering from autoimmune diseases, may already have a compromised gut that will need special attention. You can start with the diet laid out in the pillars and see how things improve. If you don't see results you like, you might try a more committed approach, like an elimination diet, an anti-inflammatory diet, the specific carbohydrate diet, or another more intensive regime.

Ideally you should work with someone who can help you on this front, like a good Functional Medicine or integrative doctor or health coach, but I'll give you a short "nutshell" summary here of the most common approach that any good doctor will start with, the *elimination diet*. An elimination diet typically removes foods that are known troublemakers from your diet for at least thirty days. This timeframe may vary; some practitioners feel twenty-one days is enough, while others say two months. This is usually enough time for your immune system to calm down. Once it has, you can reintroduce foods one at a time to see how your body responds.

This process helps folks get to the bottom of what foods are causing their symptoms. Everyone is unique. Some people react to certain foods, while others are fine with them. You have to investigate to see which foods work better or worse for you. Doing so can help you feel much better. You may even be surprised at how some foods are negatively impacting you.

While there are many foods that could cause trouble in your gut, the top known offenders are:

- Gluten (a protein in wheat and some other grains)
- Dairy (particularly the protein called *casein* and the sugar called *lactose*)
- Eggs
- Soy
- Corn
- Nightshades (tomatoes, eggplant, peppers)
- Beans and Legumes
- And of course, sugar, refined flours and carbs, and bad fats—all listed in Pillars 2 and 3.

Most elimination diets start with this list and have you remove all items, with nightshades and beans/legumes being more negotiable. Caffeine and alcohol are two other items you want to avoid. After the time period you choose, you can reintroduce each food, one at a time, to see which one(s) might be causing your challenge(s). You need to wait four days after a reintroduction before reintroducing another food, as many symptoms are actually delayed in the body. If a food is good, you can keep that one in your diet and then re-introduce the next one on the list. If you feel symptomatic, then take that item back out for another few weeks and try it again later to see if staying off of it will help it clear.

The good news is that over time, as you continue to heal and your inflammatory immune response calms down, you can sometimes reintegrate persistently symptomatic foods into your diet. Some sadly may not make the cut for the long haul, but you'll find plenty of delicious and workable alternatives.

Again, I recommend working through this process with a professional. If this is not an option for you, there are some good self-guided protocols you can check out. See my references section at the end for suggestions.

Gut Disorders: IBS, SIBO, Crohn's Disease, Ulcerative Colitis, and Celiac Disease

Gut disorders and diseases sure can be problematic. I've been challenged with what is called post-infectious IBS for almost thirty years, and it's been no easy ride. For those with conditions like Crohn's disease, ulcerative colitis, celiac disease, the pillars within this book will likely help, as all of them are essential for any respectable healing diet. However, keep in mind that you will likely need a very specialized diet due to your condition, and should try to work with a specialized healthcare professional to determine what that diet is. Again, I'd highly recommend a Functional Medicine, integrative or naturopathic doctor.

The good news is that many of these conditions can be calmed and very often even reversed. You can look at diets like Specific Carbohydrate, Low FODMAP

(especially for IBS and SIBO), and GAPS to help calm your system and begin the healing process. A good elimination diet, as described just previously, is a core feature for each of these. You can Google the diets mentioned to learn more about each of them. There are many online courses and even online health coaches that can help guide you through the diets.

Digestive Bitters and Enzymes

The body produces a whole host of enzymes to help us break down food in the digestive tract. Various enzymes are secreted in your mouth the moment you take your first bite or sip and secretions occur all the way through the digestive system. Many foods also contain enzymes. As we age, most of us lose at least some of our capacity to produce these digestive enzymes ourselves, inhibiting our ability to properly break down food, which makes the nutrients less available for proper absorption.

A poor-quality Standard American Diet can make our lack of enzymes an even more pronounced issue. If you have digestive challenges like chronic constipation or diarrhea, gas, bloating, acid reflux, or other related issues, chances are good you don't have enough enzymes at work. While there can be a number of other contributing factors to these kinds of digestive challenges, unbalanced enzymes are often at play as well.

Many Functional Medicine, naturopathic and Integrative practitioners will encourage people suffering these symptoms to supplement their diet with enzymes to help maximize digestion and nutritional absorption. There are a variety of enzymes that do different things and help digest specific kinds of foods. If you work with an integrative oriented practitioner, they can order urine and blood tests that can help determine which enzymes you are most in need of.

Alternatively, you can try a broad-spectrum enzyme to give yourself a general boost. The good news for most is that as you shift to a healthier diet, over time, your body will likely start to produce more enzymes again. If you do try supplementing enzymes, start low and go slow. Your body may not be used to these enzymes and you may need an adjustment period.

Another good alternative or even simultaneous option is to take digestive bitters right before eating (20-30 minutes ahead of time is ideal). These bitters help stimulate your body's own production of natural enzymes as well as kick start the digestive process. Urban Moonshine is a brand I like. They make a variety of enzymes with different herbs that are very stimulating. When I work with anyone with digestive issues, this is usually where we start.

Bone Broth

Bone broth is being rediscovered as a superfood, particularly for its gut-healing strengths. I say rediscovered because our ancestors, recent ones at that, used bone broth as a regular dietary staple (many still do in various parts of the world), but it fell out of favor in the West as our busy modern lives and addictions to quick processed foods have taken hold. You may have heard about it of late as it's gaining a lot of steam in the nutrition community and is becoming a more mainstream health food.

The name turns some off, but it's really just a glorified broth with far more benefits. In addition to gut health, it's great for your skin, joints, organs, hair, eyes, metabolism, immune system, hydration, and much more. There are many good individual components within it, including gut-healing amino acids. Collagen is also a praised nutrient in bone broth, which is a building block for healthy skin, joints, and more. As we age, most of us lose our capacity to produce collagen internally as well as we could in our youth, and we need to be careful to replenish this through our diet.

You can make bone broth yourself pretty easily. I like to use a crock pot, but the stove is fine, too. To make it, simply slow-cook all the bones and cartilage that are left over from your meats. Use a large container and let it gently boil for at least twenty-four hours, or up to forty-eight. This slow-cooking method helps all the gelatin, collagen, marrow, amino acids, and other minerals and nutrients leach into the broth.

Fill up your pot with water, a tablespoon of apple cider vinegar, and put in bones and joints from whatever leftovers you have. (As always, try to use bones from organic, pasture-raised or grass-fed animals.) You want to fill the pot about a third of the way with bones and joints. They could come from something like a whole chicken you used for a soup. Many markets now sell frozen bones and joints just for making bone broth; you can always ask your butcher if you don't see them in the meat department of your grocery store.

For flavoring, you can add in vegetables, herbs, and salt as you would with a regular broth. You want to skim the fat off the top when it's done, as the longer cooking times can cause some oxidation to the fat lipids. Finally, strain the broth out and compost the bones and physical matter.

You can freeze the broth for long-term use. Add it to soups, use it to make sauces, or drink it like tea in a cup, as many cultures still do. A cup a day is generally considered plenty. Freezing it in an ice cube tray is one option, then transfer to a ziplock and you can grab them out of the freezer when you need them.

You can also find premade bone broth in most health food stores and some mainstream ones. Kettle and Fire or Epic are good brands.

If you are not Vegan or Vegetarian, I'd strongly urge you to research bone broth benefits for yourself and to consider making it a staple in your diet. Just a cup a day can go a long way to help keep the doctor away.

Eliminating Gluten

You likely saw gluten listed earlier in the elimination diet and I talked about it briefly earlier in the book. Gluten is one of the more problematic substances in food that we are exposed to in the Standard American Diet. Gluten is simply a class of proteins that occur in many grains, wheat being the most common source. For most of human evolution, we didn't eat the kinds of gluten we are exposed to now. Frankly, we didn't eat a lot of grains to begin with in many cultures. But as the agricultural revolution took hold and we started to eat more grains, we also learned to hybridize them and change their molecular makeup to be more profitable to mass produce. This newer, hybridized gluten has been particularly problematic in terms of its impact on our health, creating many negative consequences.

A small percentage of the population, less than one percent, have full blown celiac disease. If one has this disease and eats even the tiniest amount of gluten, it can cause significant damage to the intestines. It's a very serious and acute autoimmune disease. Additionally, a growing number of digestion researchers and experts think that somewhere between forty and sixty percent of the population, while not celiac, are gluten intolerant or sensitive. Intolerances can also damage the lining of your intestines and lead to a whole host of problems, as described in the gut health section previously. It's important to be aware of this. I typically urge everyone to at least try to get off gluten and see how they feel. I don't eat it myself and have found it to be a particularly problematic food when I've done elimination diets and retested it.

But please be mindful when getting off gluten that many of the gluten-free alternatives are still not part of a healthy diet. They are typically full of refined carbs and sugars.

If you'd like to learn more about why gluten can be so challenging on the body, I'd encourage you to check out a great overview article from Paleo Leap here: http://bit.ly/2GFHCIB.

Dairy Challenges

Dairy can also be a pretty complicated food for many to handle. This is particularly true due to the dairy-based protein called casein, which I mentioned previously. A significant percentage of the population often unknowingly has a hard time processing this particular protein, and their intolerance to it can cause immune dysregulation and even chronic low-level inflammation.

Some people who are challenged by dairy can tell right away, with symptoms flaring up soon after eating, but it can take days after eating it for others to feel symptoms.

Many people also have a problem with a dairy sugar called lactose. While there are enzymes one can take to help better process the lactose, there is not much that can be done with casein. One good piece of news is that butter has very little casein and not much lactose, so most tolerate it better than milk or cheese. Hard, aged cheeses also have lower amounts of lactose for those that have a problem with it.

You can test your body and see how you react by removing dairy from your diet for twenty one to thirty days as described in the elimination diet. Then see how you feel when you start back again. If you don't feel well after re-introducing, it might be smart to skip it and find better alternatives as much as possible. I have found that raw goat cheese and goat milk are more tolerable for me, and I've used goat milk in recipes that call for cow's milk. Again, you will have to see how your unique body reacts.

Mindful Eating

Healthy eating is about more than just what you put in your mouth. It's also *how* you allow it in. *Mindful eating* includes chewing slowly, breathing deeply, and allowing space between bites. This greatly aids in proper digestion and helps us better absorb nutrients.

The *vagus nerve*, located at the back of your head, is one of the strongest regulators of good digestion and is very easily impacted by stress. Another reason to eat slowly and as calmly as possible, with plenty of breathing time, is that it helps the vagus nerve function better. Eating "on the run" or shoveling it down will have consequences, so be mindful.

For those of you into such things, I try to make the eating process a kind of spiritual practice. When I'm doing so, I visualize the nutrients that are flooding into my body spreading around and nourishing every cell. I bless the food before I eat it, giving thanks to all the workers, plants, animals, and mechanisms that were at play to get this food to me. Every bite can be a moment to breathe and stay present and conscious of the food and its nourishment.

I think it is important to be present to and visualize a higher purpose for ourselves and our bodies, to be connected to what will allow us to thrive. That way, when we make our food choices, as with any life choice, we are in tune with what our bodies really want and need to serve our life's purpose, to serve our joy.

Chewing

Speaking of chewing, did you know that your mouth releases important digestive enzymes called *amylase* and *lipase* which help kick off the body's digestive process? Chewing properly not only starts the process of food breakdown from our teeth gnashing, but also bathes the foods in the enzymes longer, aiding the entire downstream digestive process.

The process of chewing properly also helps eliminate bloating, gas, and abdominal pain. Needless to say, chewing is an important part of nutrition that too many of us don't pay much attention to as we rush through eating in response to our frenzied, busy lives.

When we combine mindful eating and take the proper time to chew, we can also impact our weight. This combination triggers signals that tell the brain when the body is properly satiated and doesn't need more food.

A good rule of thumb is to try to chew each bite at least twenty-five times, adjusting this number depending on how tough or raw a food is. This may be way outside your norm, but it can be an important and manageable part of better health.

Indigestion

Indigestion is a pretty good sign we are not eating what we should be. It means that our digestive system and its supportive enzymes are not able to keep up with the load that has been introduced. Common culprits are coffee, sweets, fried foods, and alcohol.

Two of my favorite treatments for indigestion are the herbs parsley and ginger. I personally find parsley to be the most effective. It quells a sour stomach quicker and more effectively than anything, even over-the-counter drugs.

If you tend to pop an antacid to cure your indigestion, I would encourage you to stop. Antacids, especially acid blockers, can really screw up our delicate digestive systems and create long-term consequences. They mess with our natural enzyme production and squelch stomach acid production, which is often under-producing already.

Cooking Power Tips: *Let Cooking be an Enjoyable Experience; Making the Best Use of Time to Prepare Delicious and Healthy Foods*

Cooking can be a very fun and enjoyable experience. Since food is literally the life sustaining energy for our bodies, I try to keep perspective on how important it is to my own life and vitality. As much as I'm able, I allow myself to get in a good groove with cooking, and even have fun with it!

Cooking can be a mindful experience, sometimes even meditative. I try to savor it, make it a process of slow, sustainable living that I can enjoy and use to wind down. I like to smell the fragrances, be in the flow of what is needed in the preparation process. It can really be fun and enlivening when I sync up with my cooking ritual. I sometimes add a glass of wine to spice it up (although this sometimes ramps up my anxiety when cooking a big meal with lots of multitasking).

It's also great to cook with a friend, partner, child, or other loved one. Make it a collaborative and creative exercise. This helps cut down on cook time and can be a chance to bond and connect. Set your intentions beforehand and plan out your meal so that any risk of tension can be minimized and instead transformed into quality time.

I know some people feel like they aren't cut out for cooking, or are even outright disdainful of the idea. I urge you to give it a heartful try. Put on some good music, maybe even catch up on a TV show to distract yourself. If I'm not making cooking a mindful exercise, I like to put on something mindless and cheesy, like a reality singing competition show… (Stop judging!) It's also a good time to listen to an audio book or a podcast.

When we cook, we have full control of what ingredients we put into our bodies. We can control quality and maximize nourishment. I believe the effort pays off, and as a result, I make sure I'm having a creative, enjoyable time as often as possible.

Time Management

I'm all too aware of the challenges many face when it comes to cooking, especially when one has a busy life. It can be tricky or feel impossible at times. Here are some tricks to help you prepare and manage a better balance.

First off, and this may seem obvious, plan out your meals for the week. The more organized you are, the better your time management will be. Many people do their shopping for the week on Sundays. They create their master meal plans, shopping lists, and get all their loot. Sundays are also a good time to do food pre-prep. If you need to for a busy week ahead, you can clean and even chop vegetables, etc., for various meals.

Another great way to save time is to use a grocery delivery service. To start, Google "grocery delivery" options as well as "community supported agriculture" in your city. Amazon Pantry exists in many places, and now helps customers use Whole Foods health food stores, but there are other options in most cities. One of my favorite services is Thrive Market, an online organic retailer. They provide high-quality health foods and lots of fun treats and snacks that aren't as bad as mainstream versions, at good prices. Their products are shipped, so they don't do fresh foods, but they do have loads of staples.

You can do all your shopping online, save your favorites, and make your life that much easier. I live in

Oakland, California, where we have a service called Good Eggs, which is fresh food sourced from local farmers. You may have a similar service in your area.

If you'd like even more help, there are now some really creative apps to help you with all the steps, from recipes to food delivery. The **Real Plans app** is one to look at. It does more than plan your meals. It gets to know your family's likes and dislikes. Remembers your favorite recipes. Tracks your macros. Streamlines shopping. And will even get groceries delivered to your doorstep. You can choose different diets as well. (The "Paleo" option is closest to the information laid out here, but they have other healthier choices too, including vegetarian.) You can learn more at www. realplans.com.

Instant Pot/Pressure Cookers

Go get an Instant Pot (or other brand of a pressure cooker) ASAP! These really are little miracles for quick and easy cooking. If you haven't heard of them, Instant Pots are high-pressure cookers that can cook foods at light speed while maintaining good nutrients. A chicken that might take an hour to roast in the oven is done in twenty-five minutes in my Instant Pot and still tastes good! Tender and juicy, too. The same goes for a pot roast or brisket. Squash, carrots, sweet potatoes, so many things can get done quickly and taste good. Soups are perfection—something about the pressurization seems to infuse the ingredients with the flavors and herbs I add in. Curry dishes are great too. You just toss all the ingredients in, close the lid, hit start and it's all done for you from there!

There are now entire websites and Instant Pot cookbooks with recipes out there to give you loads of creative ideas. To get started, check out Nom Nom Paleo's cookbooks at www.nomnompaleo.com.

Mason Jar Salads

In Pillar 3, I mentioned mason jar salads as a good way to indulge in vegetables. This is a clever idea that you can find more info about all over the web. It works great for lunches at work when you want to eat healthy but have fewer options than you do at home.

Sold on the idea? Here's how you do it. Take a large mason jar, and pack it full of healthy ingredients. You can fill up several for the week all at the same time. They are easy to carry around and fit nicely in the fridge. Many recipes use the thirty-two-ounce jars, but I like a lot of salad, so I go for larger!

- Step 1: Put in your dressing first. You want your moist elements (like tomatoes) at the bottom of the jar so that pre-prepped salads don't get soggy.
- Step 2: Anything heavy or big is next. Put in your protein, grain, beans or chopped veggies and fruit.
- Step 3: Add extra items like nuts, seeds, dried fruits, or anything you want to stay dry.
- Step 4: Your leafy greens. These need to be at the top so they are kept dry until right before eating. You don't want them wilting away.

You can compress your items in the jar. Right before eating, shake it up to get all those good fats in the dressing at the bottom to spread around and coat the entire salad. Remember to try and let the oil sit on your colorful lettuce and greens for ten minutes if you can, as it makes the nutrients more bioavailable. You can then eat your salad straight out of the jar or enjoy it in a large bowl.

Power Tip: I use stainless steel lids with a silicone insert for my reusable mason jar "projects" (salad dressings, storage, etc.). That way, my food gets minimal exposure to toxins from plastics, like BPA. See "Environmental Toxins: Get Rid of the Plastics" for more info on toxins to avoid.

Sheet-Pan Meals

Another great way to easily and quickly prep meals is to cook your whole meal on a sheet pan (i.e. a cookie sheet). You can pre-cut and prep items at the start of your week, then spread it out on a single cookie sheet and bake it in your oven at the same time: meat, vegetables, starches, and all. Use Google to find many great recipes. The *Real Food Dietitians* have thirty paleo-oriented sheet-pan meals here: http://bit.ly/2OPHIEC.

Paleo Meal Delivery Services

If you can afford it, there are now many health-conscious meal delivery services. Some have the whole meal cooked, others do the prep work and then you cook. You will have to Google to find out what is available in your area, but one way to help is to use a term like "paleo," which will target higher-quality services that fit the four pillars better.

Eating Good Food More Affordably

If money is an issue, you can read tips on how to make healthy eating more affordable here: http://bit.ly/3l97kbV and http://bit.ly/2PPZrfK or http://bit.ly/2OQZYxn.

Proper Hydration: *Water is a Life Force; Get Plenty to Keep your Body in Proper Flow*

Proper hydration is critical for health. Up to sixty percent of the adult human body is actually water, so keeping it all fresh, flowing, and replenished is important.

Unfortunately, most of us do not drink enough water. Some medical surveys have shown that sixty to seventy percent of us don't drink the required amounts of water daily. I'm sorry to say, folks, but coffee, soda, and juice are not the best sources of hydration! Too much of those liquids will deplete your body of important electrolytes like potassium, in addition to the problems mentioned earlier regarding sugar.

Drinking plenty of filtered water helps us flush toxins out of our bodies through our kidneys and intestines. It helps lubricate our joints, helps transport nutrients around the body, keeps our digestion flowing properly, and much more. Dehydration can not only make us physically unwell—it's a big cause of headaches, for example—it can also mess with our mental health and emotions. For so many reasons, make sure you are drinking liquids adequately.

Water really is the best source of hydration, and filtered water is ideal. It's very important to drink filtered water as most municipal systems not only don't filter out all the toxins, they often add them in! Chlorine and fluoride are only two of the many worrisome chemicals added. These added toxins go straight into the body and can have a whole host of consequences. Read more in the section "Minimizing Environmental Toxins" that follows for tips on the best kinds of filters to look for. Be sure also to drink out of glass or uncoated metal, as plastics leach a whole host of toxins you don't want to add into your water.

Flat water is great. If you don't have digestive issues, bubbly water can be good, too. Vegetables and fruits also contain a good amount of water and have balancing electrolytes, like potassium, calcium, sodium, magnesium, and other minerals that are critical elements to keep us hydrated.

If you work out heavily or have chronic dehydration issues, you can also add electrolyte powders to your water to get an extra boost. Filtering water can remove many of the electrolyte minerals, so these can also help there. Just make sure to get a version that doesn't contain sugar (or bad "fake" sugars)—as clean as you can find. A pinch or two of high-quality sea salt can also be added to water to increase its hydrating capacity and electrolytes (this is what I use).

How much water you should drink each day can depend on a number of factors, like your weight, the weather (e.g., heat requires more), and how much exercise you are getting, as sweating depletes electrolytes. As with food, each body is unique, and our own hydration needs are unique. Certainly we want to drink plenty of water when we are thirsty. That is the number one sign that it's past time for more liquid, or that you might be starting to get dehydrated.

Many health experts suggest we aim for about half our body weight in ounces each day, which averages out to about six to eight ten-ounce glasses per day. On the higher end of the scale, some experts recommend that men intake around 100 ounces (or twelve cups, of measured liquid) and women about 70 (nine measuring cups). That's quite a range of suggestions! Pay attention to your body when you drink water, and try out drinking more and less to see how it impacts you. Don't overdo it either (don't worry, most of you aren't!), you can flush out too many electrolytes if you go too far overboard.

One alternative to counting cups of water per day is to watch the color of your urine. Generally speaking, urine of a lighter color means you are getting adequate water. The darker yellow it is, the less hydrated you are. This is a sign that your cells are shrinking and trying to preserve water stores. This isn't 100% foolproof, but can be considered a helpful rule of thumb.

Good news, though: if you are eating plenty of vegetables and fruit as described earlier in the book, you are getting about twenty percent of your hydration through them and other high-liquid foods.

If you are one of the many folks who say they have a hard time remembering to drink water, try setting reminders on your smartphone throughout the day, or think of something that happens frequently, like getting a text message or an email alert, as a reminder to take a sip (or better yet, a swig).

And if you are one of the people who say they don't like the taste of water (I really don't get this since it's flavorless, but I've heard it from quite a few folks so it's got to be true), try adding a squeeze of lemon or lime to give it a bit of flare. I also like to use a splash of pure lower-sugar cranberry juice (not the sweetened variety). There are also special pitchers out on the market that have compartments for putting in fruit or herbs to soak and flavor the water (e.g. cucumber, mint). All of these options work great with chilled bubbly water, too, for a fresh and tasty beverage that is much better than sugary soda.

I always start my day with a large glass of water to kick-start my good health. It's a great way to flush out the toxins that have accumulated and been processed by the body overnight. I start my day feeling hydrated, more buoyant, and ready to roll. Try drinking more liquids and see how you feel. Your body will likely thank you.

The Psychology of Change: *How to find the inner motivation to achieve your goals successfully*

Almost any kind of change can take time, especially when we are trying to change deeply entrenched patterns. It's important when making big dietary shifts to be honest with yourself and set realistic goals. When we overshoot we tend to miss our mark and then get disheartened for future efforts. Taking on too much too quickly is a surefire way to disappointment. Pushing our limits to some degree is a good thing, but overstretching them can cause trouble.

First, be gentle with yourself. Celebrate even the small victories. When you miss a mark, don't be too hard on yourself. Get back on track and continue to make improvements.

Let's face it, changing diet and lifestyle is not always easy. We have years of entrenched habits to attend to. It can be emotional on many levels, and everyone is unique in how they handle change. It's not just psychological either, it's also physiological. We get wired into habits, and our bodies get used to patterns. Don't sweat it too much if change is hard at first. If you really feel like you can't handle it, pull back a little and step in more slowly.

Time is definitely a friend on this front. For many of us, as we make adjustments, even minor ones, we start to get used to them and they become our new norms.

I remember when I started a deeper plunge into a healthier diet, there were many moments that were hard. There were so many times I didn't think I could pull it off. But in time, I adjusted and then new tastes and sensations became my norm. Things I didn't think were satiating before became so. Flavors that I didn't initially like started to become not just tolerable; they became delicious and even preferable. A big mistake I think I made was that I went too fast, felt like I needed to reach my highest goals immediately and it caused unnecessary stress.

You might feel hopeless that you can't enjoy food like you once did, but if you commit to these pillars, you'll likely discover that you have opened up a whole new world of enjoyment. The flavors and tastes of cheap, processed foods, especially sugars, will start to taste overwhelming or downright bad. I cannot handle the levels of sugar I once did, and in cutting back, I can now appreciate so many other flavors and elements of food. My taste buds have awoken from a long deprivation and slumber!

Eating and living well are one of the ultimate acts of self-love, something of which we are all in short supply.

Get Support

One of the most important things you can do to help make a lasting change is to get support. Community is the best way to form new habits and get healthy. If you can enlist a friend or two to join you, or a significant other, this support can make you both far more successful.

There are other means of support as well. You can find online support groups on places like Facebook or go to Meetup.com to find in-person groups. Search online for other communities of support. Try using words like "paleo diet" in your search, as people who follow this diet are more closely aligned to the principles in this book.

You could also hire a health coach to work with you, either individually or in a group setting. Research shows this to be one of the most effective ways to stick to change. The camaraderie and support can be invaluable. Plus, with a health coach, you'll get loads of good ideas.

A good health coach isn't there to make you do what they want, they are there to support and guide you in your own goals and desires. You can step into these kinds of shifts at the pace and with the focus you most desire. A good Functional Medicine health coach may be best. You can also look for coaches trained in specialty areas like the paleo or anti-inflammatory diet.

Healthy Lifestyle Tips

Food nutrition is not the only thing we need to focus on for a healthy life. There are many other critical ways we need to nourish ourselves. In this section we will explore some other important factors to consider for a healthy lifestyle.

If you remember earlier in the book when I discussed epigenetic factors that drive health, you might recall that I was talking about what a powerful influence food choices have on how our good and bad genes turn on and off and drive positive or negative outcomes. The kinds of "lifestyle and environmental" factors I will discuss below can be just as influential on your health as food. Every body is different and our exposures to various toxins can have different effects on us. So it can be important to make positive changes in the variety of areas I discuss in this section as well as the food choices. The data and suggestions are all evidence-based. I'd urge you to give all of this serious consideration.

Again, this information is not exhaustive, but provides an overview of good tips to get you rolling.

- **Emotional wellness and stress reduction:** exploring the impacts of stress and emotional challenges, as well as how to better cope and cultivate more calm.
- **Minimizing household and environmental toxins:** the dangers lurking in household chemicals, personal care products, environmental toxins, and how to protect yourself.
- **Sunlight nutrients:** why you need to make sure to get enough light for good health.

- **Movement and exercise:** keep yourself moving to maximize vitality and strength.
- **The healing power of sleep:** cultivating a better sleep rhythm for optimal energy and continual healing.
- **Our collective needs:** building resilient community and working for social change.

Emotional Wellness, Stress Reduction and Healing Life's Traumas: *Exploring the Impacts of Stress and Emotional Challenges, How to Better Cope and Cultivate More Calm*

It's probably no surprise that too much stress is not good for your health. In addition to managing stress, there are other emotional pillars that we need to strengthen in order to maintain good overall health. For many, emotional well-being can have as big an impact on physical health as any other factor. For almost all of us, it plays an important role at some level.

It's important to do stress-relieving activities and practices, attend to any childhood or adult traumas, build a strong supportive community and family, and to incorporate mindfulness into our daily lives. In this section, we will lightly explore all of this.

Stress is one of the most universal of the emotional challenges. There isn't anyone who escapes it, in fact it's a normal part of life. It is only really an issue when there is too much, unmanaged—then it can have negative effects on our health. The negative effects though are significant and for some people, a main driver of health challenges and even disease.

Chronic stress is the biggest challenge. It's those everyday stressors we experience, like: parenting responsibilities or struggles; work issues; dealing with health challenges; trying to get through school; paying all the bills at the end of the month; caring for a sick or dying loved one; and so many more that most of you reading this will probably be all too familiar with, at least where your own areas of stress rear their head. Chronic, unmanaged stress can throw your adrenal system into whack and lead to an unbalanced immune system and inflammation— which as we discussed earlier is one of the issues in our body that can cause disease. Over time, the neurons in your brain can also re-wire your brain systems, in line with the chronic stress, keeping the pattern even more entrenched.

We can't avoid stress altogether, but we can and must find ways to cultivate more calm, helping to mitigate its negative impacts. Ideally, we want to feel like life is working with us most of the time, not against us. We want to be able to either make changes to reduce stress, and/or learn to meet our challenges with more ease and buoyancy. The good news is, there is indeed a lot we can do to help turn tricky non-supportive patterns around. There are many possibilities for consideration that follow, which might be of great help to you.

Stress is one big bucket. Another mental health realm is related to "traumas" we might have had in our lives that can lead to more susceptibility for rampant stress in life or it might impact how effectively we deal with stress or conflict when it's in front of us. Traumas can be one of the drivers behind how we deal with or are impacted by challenges in life.

In my adult life and career I have studied and worked in fields related to psychology, trauma and other interconnected areas. My undergrad and post grad studies focused on these fields. My career, prior to and concurrent with my work on nutrition, has been spent researching certain aspects of the human condition related to trauma and working for policy advocacy relating to it all. I've learned a lot about why and how we experience our emotions and the impact they have on us, both individually and collectively, especially when sustained negative life events stunt our capacities to healthily deal with it all. While we certainly all experience stress in our lives, many people have also experienced some level of trauma as well that can be closely tied to it. There are extreme forms of trauma that some of us have faced, like severe PTSD from extreme situations, such as living in a war-torn region, living in a violent neighborhood, blunt force injuries (particularly to the head), suffering extreme child abuse or neglect, or being a victim of rape, to name a few examples.

But there are also less acute issues that are still forms of trauma, which may include any combination of things like: being bullied in school; losing a parent early in life; feeling the pressures of sexism, racism, homophobia and/or toxic masculinity; not being allowed to show or share emotions and feelings when growing up (and feeling uncomfortable or inadequate to now); not receiving enough physical affection from a safe adult as a child; or countless other real and tangible adversities that can leave their mark, especially when one has faced multiple forms. It's not just stuff from our past, current life issues can leave their mark as well.

Some would say, "Well, don't we all have these kinds of experiences to one degree or another? Isn't it just part of life? Is it really trauma?" Yes, for many people it is, and that is the bigger point. So many of us have some kind of emotional "baggage" in our closet. As social science continually better understands all this, depending on the severity and/or length of exposure, these challenging life events are now being seen as traumas, as they literally have an affect on our brain chemistry and its wiring that can be lasting and get entrenched. We can be impacted by these experiences even long after they happen. Thankfully many people had good enough experiences growing up, had plenty of love, and maybe had more limited exposures to adversity. But for those that might have had significant challenges, know that there are many people working on these issues and how to heal from them. It's worth the effort to attend to them for more positive impacts on your health and wellbeing.

When we experience any kind of trauma, large or small, especially as children, and don't have the kind of emotional support to heal from it, our brain starts to rewire itself around the experiences and the actions we take for self-protection and self-preservation. In the field of psychology, these are often called *defense mechanisms*. They can be life-saving when we are kids. As children, we cannot do much to protect ourselves when we don't have strong enough adult support systems to protect us. However, the things we had to do to protect ourselves back then can be the very things that keep us from living vibrant, emotionally fulfilled lives as adults. When wired for the traumas we have faced, our brains can make stress and anxiety hard to kick as we age and are better able to actually protect ourselves. We are still in some of the psychological patterns we were in as children who couldn't protect ourselves. This is all generational too, we pass these patterns down from one generation to the next. In the best of cases each generation does some work and improves on the last, and it can indeed be a real collective evolutionary progress forward. I believe this is what is predominantly happening and we are seeing positive collective shifts, at least in certain parts of the world.

There are huge red flags as well though. This whole cycle, especially when extreme and systemic, is likely what causes most of our human conflicts and even wars. People are still living with severe, unmitigated traumas, and "acting out" in sometimes horrific ways. There is no "mass shooter" or murderer, to name a couple of extreme examples, who isn't severely traumatized in some way that has gone out of control, whose needs weren't met by family or society and tended to by doing restorative and reparative work (or better yet, prevented when possible, which I'll talk a lot more about at the end of the book). This isn't to simply justify, or to say everyone with trauma acts out like this, but if we hope to move out of these horrible patterns, we need to better understand and begin to name what is really happening at the deeper levels and ensure supports are available.

Ultimately, when we have the tools and support to deal with these challenges—both individually and collectively—they can be growth opportunities for our individual emotional evolution. But it does take conscious, committed attention, work and healing support to "rewire" our brains for health and well-being. The neurons that have been trained to experience over-amplified stress, anxiety, depression, etc. can be shifted. You can begin to make needed shifts in your life to reduce stress and to calm down the impacts of traumas. Doing so can bring great relief.

I've been on a personal growth journey for many years, working hard to cultivate as much emotional wellness as I can for myself. I've experienced and felt firsthand the many benefits of shoring up my emotional well-being. Anxiety was one of my biggest emotional challenges. It was crippling at times. In many ways I have been blessed in my life, I had a lot of love growing up and have cultivated it in my adult life too, but I've also had some challenges and even traumas in my life that I continue to work through. I'm more than sure that some of the autoimmune challenges I'm still grappling with were at least in part stoked by these anxieties and challenges. As I've worked to calm them down, I've seen my health, vitality, and joy rise beyond what I was even sure it could. I'm so much more connected to what I'm feeling and needing and able to really stay much more in tune with what my whole self requires to be vibrant and healthy. I'm so glad to say that my life feels deeply fulfilling, adventurous, fun and so much more at peace. It is so worth every effort I've made to bring me to this place. And I look forward to what is to come as I continue!

Following are some of the paths you might consider if you feel like you fall into the bucket of categories above. Again, I won't go into great detail here, but instead will give you some key highlights and resources for further exploration. If something piques your interest, check it out. You are worth it!

Therapy

Establishing a relationship with a good therapist can be one of the most beneficial things you do to support your sustained emotional well-being if you are feeling any external life challenges or unease, and especially those feeling the effects of chronic stress of life traumas. A good therapist—whether an attachment-based therapist, a psychiatrist, or one of the many other good forms—can help you figure out what the biggest limitations are in your life and what might be most beneficial for your healing.

There are many schools of thought and forms of therapy. Everyone has their own unique needs and one form might be a better fit for some than others. The only way to know for sure what would work best for you is to learn a little

about them and then try something out that feels resonant to see. Psychology Today has compiled a big list of different approaches, which you can explore at www.psychologytoday.com/us/types-of-therapy. But from my years of research and experience, I've discovered several approaches to therapy that are more grounded in what recent research shows to be effective, especially around trauma healing and brain re-wiring. Some of the more leading-edge styles of therapy come from the attachment-based, somatic, neuroscientific, trauma-informed communities, internal family systems therapy, and/or accelerated experiential-dynamic psychotherapy (AEDP). Therapists who are trained in these emerging styles tend to be better equipped to give you what you need to build up new emotional capacities and rewire your brain for emotional health. That doesn't mean there aren't many other good approaches and therapists. Harvard has a list of questions you can ask when interviewing a potential therapist:
https://www.health.harvard.edu/depression/10-questions-to-ask-when-choosing-a-therapist

Some of the key experts I respect in these areas are Bessel van der Kolk, Diane Poole Heller, Peter A. Levine, Stan Tatkin (great stuff around relationships), Daniel J. Siegel, and Rick Hanson. Check out their websites, podcasts, books, etc. to learn more. There are many others; these are just a few I've been exposed to.

You can check out the Accelerated Experiential-Dynamic Psychotherapy Institute (AEDP), which has resources as well as a directory of trained therapists that tend to be trained in the areas I just described: www.aedpinstitute.org.

Generally speaking, therapy is not a quick fix. For many of us, we are sorting through a lifetime worth of "stuff," so don't expect immediate transformation (it can bring some swift relief though). In time, you will rewire and integrate new thoughts, feelings, and behaviors, and when you sync up with a good therapist, you will likely feel some encouragement rather swiftly.

Keep in mind, though, that therapists are people, too. There are no magic bullets, and because everyone's stories and challenges are unique, it's certainly an exploration to make sure the relationship with your therapist is a good fit. I've tried out a few therapists over the years. I've taken away valuable things from all of them, but I can also say that some have been a better fit for me than others. If someone isn't helpful to you or you are not feeling a connection with them, empower yourself to move on and try someone else.

That said, it can take time to get to know one another and get into a groove. This is true of any relationship, but sometimes you just know it's not right. Give yourself space and time if you are not sure. What you do not want to do is bail on your therapist because you don't want to face your "stuff." This is another area in which to be brave. When you accept that your emotional challenges exist and begin to move through them, it can bring such sweet relief. You might feel some discomfort or even pain in a particular moment, but it will pay off in the long run.

I know many reading this may not have good mental health coverage (or any) and feel like you can't afford this kind of support. It was certainly a challenge when I was younger and pretty broke, but I found a way. I called and asked about sliding scale support and found someone who let me pay $25 a session, and when I didn't have it, let it slide. I also re-prioritized my finances and scrapped it together. There are students studying who need training hours, you could try a local university to work with one of them. I'm not saying these possibilities will work for everyone, but it's worth setting an intention and trying.

There are also some really powerful adjuncts to therapy that are showing some really remarkable results at helping to heal traumas and even PTSD. One is more readily available, it's called Eye Movement Desensitization and Reprocessing (EMDR). This is an interactive technique where a therapist directs your eye movement in a way that can help you relive triggering or traumatic memories without the as much distress as might otherwise emerge. It's been scientifically proven to be quite effective.

Another really exciting type of adjunct therapeutic intervention is happening through the use of psychedelics, like MDMA, mushrooms (psilocybin), ketamine and even LSD. MDMA in particular just recently got FDA fast track approval for testing to treat PTSD, as it's one of the most rapid and effective approaches we have ever seen for helping to stabilize and bring healing to people. In the future, as it hopefully gets fully approved, it might be effective at helping heal all kinds of traumatic past events. The other psychedelics mentioned are proving similar results and this is an area that many are excited to see emerge. Ketamine (a regular component of anesthetics) treatment is already being used to treat depression with great effect. The Multidisciplinary Approach to Psychedelics Studies is an organization leading the way on these fronts. You can learn more here: www.maps.org

Functional Psychiatry

For those suffering from more acute psychological or psychiatric challenges that have become biochemical, like entrenched depression, bipolar disorder, or schizophrenia, you might consider seeking out a psychiatrist who is trained in Functional Medicine. Functional psychiatrists are showing themselves to be more effective than their peers in that they look at full body systems to help you heal. Although they are few and far between, they are out there.

If you cannot find a functional psychiatrist or you do not want to leave a psychiatrist you have a good rapport with, you may consider doing therapy so that you and your psychiatrist are working in conjunction with a Functional Medicine practitioner. As I shared earlier in this book, psychological and psychiatric challenges can be caused by or at least exacerbated by other body systems that are off balance. Everyone is unique and causes are different, but it typically all plays a role and cross reacts at some level, so it's still important to tend to the whole garden.

Mindfulness and Meditation

Our minds are powerful creatures! As I said previously, they get wired into habits as we age, particularly in line with our life experiences, either good or bad. It's often hard to shake ourselves out of stress or bad moods, anxiety, and so on when we have literally been wired for it over many years.

Meditation and mindfulness-based practices can work wonders for many people. A plethora of encouraging evidence has already proven major improvements for even deeply entrenched challenges like depression, fibromyalgia, and gut diseases through these practices.

Research has shown that mindfulness-based activities can help with:

- Stress Reduction
- Focus
- Boosting Working Memory
- Provide Increased Cognitive Function and Flexibility
- Reducing Emotional Reactivity
- Increased Relationship Satisfaction
- And more.

There are many different forms of meditation and almost as many mindfulness-based practices. While there are a variety of definitions, they all are focused on calming your mind, helping to bring your attention to your thoughts (often a negative chatterbox), to help you notice what your brain is churning out relating to your thinking, feelings, and sensations and to bring your awareness to the present moment—often with focus on your breath. Practices can help you develop new ways of noticing and then releasing negative thoughts and of moving forward with the ability to be more calm and centered.

I have had my own positive experiences with these practices. I have a bit of ADHD, so it's not always easy for me to quiet the chatter going on in my head! Mindful meditation has proven immensely valuable to me nevertheless. I really enjoy guided meditation for my fidgety ADHD brain. Yoga is my go to daily favorite. While some wouldn't call it meditation, I do find it very mindful and calming. It has helped me learn to regulate my breath and cultivate calm. Whatever you do, you can start small and build up.

For a great overview of key practices and online resources, visit www.bit.ly/2Oslvun. There are also many useful smartphone apps with guided meditations to help you out—two of the most popular are called Headspace and Calm. I also enjoy one called Ten Percent.

Conflict Resolution: In Relationships and the Workplace

We all face conflict in life, it's inevitable. Whether it's within ourselves or in relationship to other people. But there are better ways to deal with conflict than most of us are able to. Some responses ramp up conflict and can even lead to violence (physical or emotional). But there are also processes and ways of being that can help de-escalate and meet unmet needs which can transform conflict.

As you learn more about yourself through personal growth work and maybe good therapy, you can certainly learn skills to improve your conflict mitigation proficiencies.

Nonviolent Communication (NVC) is a great conflict resolution method developed my Marshall Rosenberg. NVC teaches us how to hear and meet our own unmet needs, and those of others. The Center for Nonviolent Communication (www.cnvc.org) broadly describes it like this: "Through the practice of NVC, we can learn to clarify what we are observing, what emotions we are feeling, what values we want to live by, and what we want to ask of ourselves and others. We will no longer need to use the language of blame, judgment or domination. We can experience the deep pleasure of contributing to each others' well being." They teach you how you can bring these lofty goals into practice in your daily life and in your various forms of relationship. This work is done in personal, organizational, and even political settings.

Another tool that can be used in the workplace is through a process created by David Rock called the SCARF Model. According to a paper he wrote, SCARF stands for the five key "domains" that influence our behavior in social situations. These are:

1. **Status**: our relative importance to others.
2. **Certainty**: our ability to predict the future.
3. **Autonomy**: our sense of control over events.
4. **Relatedness**: how safe we feel with others.

5. **Fairness:** how fair we perceive the exchanges between people to be.

The model is based on neuroscience of how the brain works, specifically in terms of threat and reward responses. When we feel threatened in the workplace, it can create all kinds of problems most of us are all too familiar with. It's stifles creativity, happiness and output. This method can help people work together better and lead to all kinds of positive results. Learn more about SCARF at: https://bit.ly/2zdvNJy You can also learn more about David and his wife Lisa's work with organizations at: www.neuroleadership.com

These are just two examples. There are many other tools out there to help you navigate the inevitable conflicts that present themselves in life.

The Mindful Benefits of Yoga

Yoga is a fantastic practice to help increase calm, presence and a sense of peace. It involves a focused attention on your breath while moving your body into various positions that help open up your body systems. It is a many millennia old practice arising out of India. It is for most people a spiritual practice, though many in the West use it more as a calming and centering exercise. (There is some controversy related to this, as some see people in the West co-opting an ancient tradition, but I won't delve into that much in this book).

I am a passionate student and practice myself. It's one of my core methods to improving my sense of emotional wellbeing. While I really love yoga classes, I primarily practice it on my own at home. Depending on the day, it might be fifteen minutes or it might be a half an hour. This could certainly count as exercise, too, but the biggest benefits I get out of my home practice are in helping to calm my system down and open me up. It literally loosens up my body, but it also opens up my energy flow. I try to pay careful attention to my breath and release stress as I get into and out of my poses.

I have a few bulging discs in my back and the yoga practice has also done wonders to help ease up the pain and open things up. It helps tremendously.

Classes can be a great way to start, as you will get direct guidance from teachers. If you don't have time for classes, there are many other great resources available virtually—some free, some for nominal fees. You can look up videos on YouTube (*Yoga with Adriene* is a good channel), or connect to apps that have teachers and breakdowns of various poses to fit specific needs.

The psychological benefits of yoga are pronounced, but there are many other physiological benefits as well, including increased muscle tone and stamina. It's also been shown to be a very effective treatment for trauma and even PTSD as it helps to rewire the brain. I couldn't recommend it more highly. It has really affected my life for the better.

Binaural Beats

This practice is very interesting. It's a kind of hack for meditation. You wear earphones and listen to two tones of slightly different frequencies, one going into each ear. Research has shown that it mimics the effects of meditation on your brain. It can also enhance your own meditation practice. If you have a smartphone you can download apps and try it out. I have found this to be pretty effective at bringing me to a state of calmness. I use an iPhone app called "Brainwave."

Breathwork

Conscious *breathwork* has long been known to have substantial health benefits including relaxation and stress reduction. According to the University of Michigan School of Medicine:

> *Deep breathing is one of the best ways to lower stress in the body. This is because when you breathe deeply, it sends a message to your brain to calm down and relax. The brain then sends this message to your body. Those things that happen when you are stressed, such as increased heart rate, fast breathing, and high blood pressure, all decrease as you breathe deeply to relax.*

It's important to note that the lung is a muscle — and just like any other muscle, it can improve with targeted exercises.

There are many different ways you can do breathwork, or breathing exercises. I'll share a couple of good ones below. Sometimes, though, I just take slow, deep breaths, pulling the air deep into my belly which helps it reach all the way down your lungs into the diaphragm, letting my belly expand instead of my chest (though another option to try is after it's full in lower parts, you can then let your chest expand as well). I let myself "vibe" into the deep breathing, and visualize that each breath is literally feeding my blood and cells with oxygen and nourishment. Then I visualize breathing out CO_2 and toxins (which actually do expel through exhales), very much like the rhythm and cycle of life. I'll do this a lot when I'm doing yoga or just sitting down, in need of tapping into my calmer self.

Another practice I use is called the 4-7-8 technique (which I believe was created by Dr. Andrew Weil). It's very nice, a quick way to ground myself and bring more calm when I need it. It's very simple and involves just three steps:

1. Put your tongue on the roof of your mouth, towards the front and above your front teeth, and breathe in deep through your nose for four seconds.
2. Then hold the top of the breath to the slow count of seven.
3. Finally, exhale through your mouth slowly to the count of eight, keeping your tongue in the same place. Do this four (or more) times in a row.

"Box Breathing" works similarly but with a different twist. Instead of the 4-7-8 count, you:

1. Inhale for four counts,

2. hold your breath for four counts,
3. exhale for four counts,
4. hold your breath for four, and
5. repeat as needed.

You can Google either of these practices to learn more.

It's important to note that when I started these techniques, I found them relieving fairly early on in the practice, but it's definitely felt more pronounced the longer I've been doing them.

Tapping

According to Jessica Ortner, author of *The Tapping Solution*, "Tapping (also known as EFT) is a stress relief technique based on ancient Chinese acupressure points and modern psychology. Tapping on acupressure points while you focus on your stress is thought to send a calming response to the brain making it possible to relax.

"Harvard studies show [that] stimulating selected meridian acupoints decreases activity in the amygdala, as well as other parts of the brain associated with negative emotions. In fMRI and PET brain scans, you can clearly see the amygdala's alarm bells being quieted when acupoints are stimulated."

This practice has been championed by many as an effective tool to help calm your system down. Learn more at www.thetappingsolution.com.

Spiritual Practice

For those of you that believe in a higher power, taking on a robust spiritual practice that aligns with your values (or even better, one that tests and expands them) can prove immensely important. Whether it's through a church, a mosque, a synagogue, a temple, or your own individual practice, you can dig deeper into your purpose and find more meaning in your life.

I grew up Catholic, which certainly helped inform some of my values and beliefs. I've also explored a range of traditions and beliefs throughout my adult life. I truly wouldn't be the person I am today, and wouldn't have worked through as many issues as I have, without learning from so many worldviews. I have a deep sense of faith in something greater than myself, that I am a part of the bigger whole of all creation. I believe that love is always the best choice and a smart path forward in all my decisions. Having this anchor has helped guide and inform my choices and my sense of worth and well-being.

I have also formed community and connection around my spiritual practices and seeking. Having a loving community around you is another critical indicator of health throughout your life.

You may already have a spiritual or religious practice. Even if you do, all the above "tools" can be an important addition to your emotional toolbox. Be mindful, though, of any need for additional psychological and emotional work. There is a popular term called *spiritual bypass* that is used when someone puts on a little more sunshine and rainbows than might be real for them in a particular moment, bypassing what is really going on. Sometimes we have to be with our darkness, let ourselves experience it and let it wash through us for the light to really shine through and do the cleansing work that is needed. Trauma and emotional scars are real, and need an array of modalities to help them heal. Sometimes our faith alone can't carry us far enough when we aren't tending to emotional wounds through things like therapy.

I have a list of resources at the end of the book with practices, books, and people who have taught me much in this area.

We are Interconnected with the Greater Whole: Spending Time in Nature

Spending time in nature is one of the most healing and restorative practices we can engage in.

In my early collegiate studies, I focused on the field of ecopsychology and learned much about the role nature plays in our psychological well-being, in fact, our deep interconnection with it. Being animals ourselves, we too are obviously a part of nature. It's not just something "out there." We evolved much more intimately in tune with the cycles and rhythms of the earth than we are now. Our very livelihood depended on us being so.

We don't seem to realize as much now, but our survival and wellbeing still very much depend on it. Too often now, nature is "out there," not a part of our daily experience. And yet the ebbs and flows of nature and life are so interconnected, even when we are disconnected from our awareness of it.

Modern, technology fueled, overly materialistic and busy lives too often disconnect us from the natural rhythms of life, especially when we don't spend time in nature nor pay enough attention to what is going on outside of our little bubbles. When we evolved there were no heated and cooled homes that isolated us from what was going on outside. Nor miles and miles of paved over, developed lands and siloed homes, offices, highways, etc. We evolved mostly in tight communities and tribes. We ate foods that were in season and understood much better the intricacies of what was happening to all other life around us. Now most of us have only a very passing connection to the greater world out there. We use technology to wrangle nature to our advantage, or at least what we think is to our advantage, but it can only go so far without consequences. And most of us give little thought to what price we pay for this new disconnected way of being and living, but there is a great cost.

We certainly see some of the negative consequences. Obviously, we have allowed environmental degradation to cause such looming catastrophes as global warming, which will be a collective challenge like humanity has never faced. We also see the ill effects that things like dirty air and water have on our health. But the disconnection also affects us on a very intimate and personal level. When we silo ourselves off from whole Earth systems thinking and understanding, we can get lodged into our own interpersonal patterns that reflect this disconnection. We can lose sight of not only what is happening to our physical planet, but also humanity, our communities, friends and family, and even ourselves. It's very important to be aware of this all and to make time and effort to stay better connected and tuned into the natural rhythms of everyone and everything on the planet and ourselves.

There are many benefits. Spending time in nature has been shown to reduce stress and to have a very calming effect on the body. Whether it's a nature hike, a walk on the beach, cultivating a garden in your yard, doing environmental justice work, or whatever appeals to you, spend more time connecting to the earth—and hopefully help take better care of it. Doing so will help calm your internal systems and connect you more deeply with the natural flow of all creation.

When we are out exploring nature, paying close attention to what is going on, allowing the sweet complexities of our planet to wash over us, we can get back in tune, to one degree or another. Being in the calm, quite, slowness of it all is a very body regulating activity.

It's important to always remember that we are not separate from the Earth and nature, we are deeply interconnected and interdependent. What we do to the Earth, we do to ourselves. Let's plug in more and take great care.

Building Family and Community

People with strong and positive connections to family, community, and/or friends have been shown to have a longer lifespan and better overall health, emotionally and physically. You may already have a lot of positive connections in your life, or you may not. Regardless, consider taking steps to build stronger connections with others.

For those without a lot of social connections, this may feel daunting, especially if you feel socially awkward. Putting yourself out there, over time, can build emotional muscles and resilience and make it easier to reach out to people as you grow. One way to take the pressure off is to look for people who share your values or passions. Find a meet-up group, join a club or church, or take a class. Even online communities can provide some support and connection.

Oh, and pets have been shown to make us more emotionally resilient as well!

For optimal health (and of course happiness) don't short-shrift your relations!

Minimizing Environmental Toxins: *The Dangers of Household Chemicals, Personal Care Products, Environmental Toxins, and How to Protect Yourself*

It's convenient and maybe even logical to think that if a product is on the market and for sale, it must be safe. Surely our government wouldn't let toxic products come into our homes, right? In the main, this is not true. There are some important standards, but as with so many actions taken by our government, the decisions are tainted by big industry lobbyists and conflicting worldviews that often ignore fairly conclusive science showing the health hazards, or at least the health risks, of a whole host of toxins.

The standards that do get set often ignore what can happen when we are exposed to multiple suspect chemicals (which we almost always are), creating even more pronounced negative effects. Researchers will often study single, specific toxins, but they don't study the accumulative exposure we get from a variety of toxins from products—that is, how they interact and ultimately accumulate inside our body over the years.

What we know, though, is that we are inundated with external toxic exposure every day from so many sources and through so many methods. One of the most respected organizations working in this space, performed a small study that detected 287 commercial chemicals, pesticides, and pollutants in the umbilical cord blood from 10 newborn infants, randomly selected by the Red Cross from U.S. hospitals. Those are disturbing numbers. I've read studies that have identified many more chemicals when you include muscle tissue and organ storage, which is where toxins go to be stored when your body is overrun and can't "detox" properly.

Even when we are exposed at low levels, these toxins can add up and cause long- and short-term damage. Our bodies were simply not designed to handle the toxic load they are being inundated with in our modern life. It's important to be mindful of this and minimize as best as we can our overall toxic burden.

You can probably imagine why it's hard to do studies on humans with such troubling chemicals, but animal studies point to some disturbing consequences.

This problem is widespread and runs deep, likely touching each of us. While we will not be able to perfectly clean up every problematic area in our own lives—and we don't want to add on top of it a build-up of stress or fear around it all—the more we can reduce our overall "toxic load," the better it will be for our long-term health. Cleaning up our lives doesn't have to be hard. There are a lot of easy things we can do and swaps we can make that are better for our health.

We've already talked about how pesticides, preservatives, and other chemicals in and on our foods can have a detrimental impact on our health, as well as the importance of going organic to help minimize our exposure to them. Following are some additional steps that can be taken to help minimize other types of toxins in the body.

Air Quality

Our lungs play a big role in toxic exposure as they can absorb pollutants through the air, spreading them quickly around our body. Given that there are many toxins floating around the air in our modern, dirty world, from factories, power plants, and automobile exhaust just to name a few, it makes sense that the quality of the air and the pollution of our daily life would play a significant role in our overall health.

It's not just outdoor air that's a problem. What many don't realize is that indoor air quality can be just as bad. Actually it's often worse than what is outside. Some research estimates that **indoor air quality can be two to five times more polluted than outside air.**

Inside the home or office, there are of course things like dust (and mites) and animal dander that can trigger allergies, but there are also other lesser-known toxins:

- Your new sofa and dresser are likely off-gassing chemicals used when processing, like flame retardants, formaldehyde, varnish, and noxious glues from the cheaply produced particle board.
- That newly painted kitchen (which I'm sure looks great!) is likely loaded with volatile organic compounds (VOCs) unless you used a low or no VOC paint.
- Water damage can create mold, bacteria, and other troubling agents.
- Mainstream cleaning chemicals that release many known irritant and toxicants.
- Low-quality air fresheners, both sprays and the plug-in variety, are loaded with troubling chemicals. Candles as well.

These and MANY other elements contain toxins that are known endocrine disrupters (which can mimic and interfere with the body's natural circulating hormones), cancer-causing agents, and respiratory irritants.

Sayer Ji, researcher and founder of Green Med Info, shares this about why cumulative exposure from multiple fronts can pose serious health risks:

As with any toxic chemicals, the amount to which we are exposed is a critical factor in health outcomes. With so many products coming together under the roof of the average home, it's a safe bet that multiple contamination sources are lurking. When these toxicants converge, not only do the overall levels of each chemical increase, but volatile organic compounds can bind with other VOCs, forming new and sometimes more dangerous compounds that are so limitless in their potential formations, it's virtually impossible to study them and ascertain their risk. Even if your favorite spray cleaner has been tested for safety and passed, it hasn't been tested for how it combines with your favorite scented lotion, which you apply several times a day. Or how it mixes with the toilet cleaner, vinyl shower curtain, soap scum remover, and Glade plugin in a tiny bathroom, where the door is usually shut. The types of emissions coming from these and other household products are serious enough to warrant concern on their own merits. The potential toxic combinations that can form should seal the deal when it comes to evaluating if these products deserve a place in your home.

— From "Consumer Alert: Air Fresheners," Green Med Info.

While outdoor air pollution is harder for most of us to address, we can and should take care inside the home and office, where we spend most of our time. There are some key things we can do to better protect ourselves.

Off-Gassing: *Let new products and furniture breathe awhile before bringing them into your home.*

I'm sure you know the smell that comes with many new products. When you first open it up, the scent (chemicals) releases right up into your nostrils. These smells aren't just harmless side effects of manufacturing. Most of them are known toxins that are often permissible by law, but less than ideal for our overall health, again, especially when you consider the accumulated load. Plus, standards shift from nation to nation, and most of our products are now made overseas, often in countries with very lax laws and/or law enforcement that make things hard to monitor well.

Many toxins will break apart and form these gases. When they are wrapped up in tight plastics, they are trapped inside the products waiting for their big escape when they reach your door and are unwrapped. Therefore, if I'm not buying green or eco-friendly products, I try to let new products—especially new furniture—off-gas outdoors before bringing into the house. Sunlight is a good accelerator of off-gassing if you can swing some full sun exposure. So, whether it's a new couch, a bedframe, or even a mattress, I suggest putting it out for up to two weeks (depending on outdoor weather). If I can't do that, I'll put it in the garage.

To determine if outdoor off-gassing will be necessary, I use the smell test to see how bad it still smells. It's not scientific, but at least I know I'm getting some of it out of the product before I bring it in and overload my lungs and body any more than necessary. I of course am always on the lookout for products that are made to be more eco-friendly, with less toxins.

Air Filters

Manually cleaning the air in your house is another smart step. We have good technology that is proven to clean up the air, at least to some degree. Everything you can do will help, so it's smart to use air filtration products in your home and office.

The following are tips for finding the healthiest air filters, according to the EWG:

- For a central air system, use a filter rated MERV 10 or higher. The higher your system can accommodate, the better it will clean.
- Clean and replace air filters regularly.
- Try out a higher-quality portable air filter. Choose one with at least a high-efficiency particulate air (HEPA) filter. You can invest more heavily and even get versions that have robust carbon filters that will filter out even more gases.
- Check the California Air Resources Board's list of certified air cleaners.

Learn more about air filtration from the EWG: http://bit.ly/2Efa2tJ.

Getting a good-quality standalone HEPA-based air filter is important as well because HEPA has the highest standards for trapping contaminants. When shopping for stand-alone filters, be sure to learn how much square footage they will filter out. Larger homes need more than one. You want the smallest micron filtration you can find for the price you can afford.

We have three in our home. I use *Consumer Reports'* rankings to determine the best one to buy. Before rating, they carefully test each of the filters for actual efficacy, and the results can be found here: www.bit.ly/2UhUVnW

Low-VOC House Paints

You are probably familiar with that "new paint smell" when you're making over a room in your house. The chemicals you smell in the paint, though, are *volatile organic compounds* (VOCs), many of which are known to be noxious and to pose health risks. There are now many house paints, for both indoor and exterior, that are either low in or contain zero VOCs. Many of them rate well in terms of quality, and you'll be pleasantly surprised after painting at how mild or even odorless they can indeed smell. I highly encourage everyone to use these paints. Prices can be comparable to regular mid- or high-range VOC paints.

You want to limit your VOCs to fifty grams or fewer per liter. You also want to avoid antifungal paints, which can contain toxic chemicals as well. Look for paints certified by Green Seal 11, which limits not only VOCs but also mercury, lead, nonylphenol ethoxylates, and other known carcinogens. Learn more good dos and don'ts from the EWG at http://bit.ly/2AQGVZB.

Are Your Candles and Air Fresheners Making You Sick?

I must admit that I'm a big candle-holic! When I was a kid in the seventies and eighties, my mom always put out tons of candles when we'd have a gathering or a party. It's one of my fondest memories as that was always our final step right before everyone came over for a visit. It was a soothing ritual and meant fun was about to kick in. I carried that torch forward (pardon the pun) and now am a big candle lighter around my house. I find it soothing, and it's a nice way to have some soft light at night before bed, or for a more "special" mojo when guests come. I know many folks do the same.

After all, our species spent millennia evolving together around an evening fire, so I think a weakness for candles is baked into our DNA. It was our time of community connection and often sacred storytelling. Those flames represent the lineage we share with thousands of generations of ancestors. There is something sacred about it to me. It creates a mood and space in my evening to tap into something a little deeper. It lets my gaze shine into spots of my inner being that want and need cool, calm, and connected energy to linger for a while. For me that little flicker can be a reminder of spirit, of connection, of my eternal spark.

Okay, sorry to now bring that energy down, but what most do not realize is how many known toxins are in typical paraffin-based candles. In fact, paraffin is a petroleum waste product that is also found in diesel fumes, yikes! When burned, paraffin-based candles emit toxic chemicals like toluene and benzene, which can contribute to health risks like cancer, common allergies, and even asthma over time. Also, some of the wicks contain a thin metal wire that burns and releases melted soot into the air. Some of these include zinc or even lead. These were supposed to be banned in the early 2000s, but can still crop up.

And then there are all the potential toxins that can go into the scented candles from fake chemical scents (see "air fresheners" in the following pages).

There are some innovative companies who use a variety of base waxes to make non-paraffin and non-toxic candles. Try them out and see which you like most! You might find them at a local health-oriented store, or you can find them online, at sites like Amazon.

For safer candle options, try:

- Soy Wax (They also last up to thirty percent longer.)
- Palm Wax (Sustainably farmed only! I find these burn about as long as a typical paraffin candle.)
- Beeswax
- Coconut Wax
- Wire-Free Wicks (Look for pure cotton or paper.)
- For scented candles, look for pure essential oils only.

Air Fresheners

Many folks also like to use air fresheners. Whether they are sprays or plug-ins, most of the mainstream brands you'll find are full of chemically crafted scents that contain numerous problematic base chemicals, including VOCs, phthalates, and formaldehyde. Learn more at Green Med Info: http://bit.ly/2zLq8aB.

The plug-in varieties sure seem convenient, but they are literally using heat to "burn" or vaporize the scent into the air, along with all these toxins. You are spreading the nastiness around your home.

Dump them and look for plug-in essential oil infusers or vapor machines. You can buy organic essential oils to your liking, and then freshen the house that way. There are many models out there that are aesthetically pleasing. It's a lot less expensive and you are actually giving yourself some nice nutrients from the essential oils. In health food or other similarly oriented stores you can also find alternative sprays that use essential oils and safer base chemicals. These are also quite effective and smell lovely.

There are effortless ways to set a nice candlelit mood and bring lovely scents into your home, while also keeping your body safer. So why take the risk?

Personal Care, Cosmetics, and Cleaning Products

Our skin is our biggest organ, and is highly absorbent. Most of us don't pay much attention to what it comes into contact with, but it's another primary method for toxins to sneak into the body. We are talking about everything from soaps to cosmetics, to perfumes and cleaning products.

It's important to be mindful of what you are putting on your skin. You may have a favorite makeup brand, but many of them use petroleum as a base and contain chemicals that are suspect at best and known toxins at worst. Remember, these things accumulate over time and interact with other chemicals and pollutants stored within your body.

Cleaning supplies can be even worse. You think all that less than ideal laundry detergent and fabric softener actually comes out of your clothes? Or that the bleachy, toxic spray cleaner you use on your counter doesn't get all over your food or rubbed on your hands? Don't kid yourself. They not only stick around to get on your skin and into your mouth, you also breathe them in when using the products and as they off-gas.

The very good news is that there are now so many companies who make safer products with quality comparable to or even better than the mainstream versions we see on the commercials everyday.

Once again, the EWG comes to the rescue here. They have two great resources to help you find better products.

EWG's Skin Deep Cosmetic Database lists thousands of personal care and cosmetic products ranked by their safety. It can be found at www.ewg.org/skindeep.

EWG's Guide to Healthy Cleaning does the same with cleaning supplies. You can find it here: www.ewg.org/guides/cleaners.

They also have a really handy app for your smartphone that lets you "scan" the barcode on products at a store to find details on how clean or toxic the product is. Check out their Healthy Living app at www.ewg.org/apps.

Water Filtration

Water, like food, can introduce toxins directly into the body. As I said earlier, the water that your city pumps to you is often full of known toxins. It's important to drink plenty of water, but make sure you filter it.

Almost everywhere I go, when I ask someone how their tap water is, they tell me that their city has the cleanest water in the nation! I typically giggle internally as I've heard it all over, and I know that of course not everyone can have the cleanest water, but also most water is pretty poor quality. If you are curious how your city ranks, you can find out more about the quality of the water in your area at the EWG's Tap Water Database: www.ewg.org/tapwater.

It's important in your home to get a quality water filter. For drinking water, preferably whole home or under the counter if you can, but if not, a good countertop model works well, too.

I know those shiny, prepackaged plastic bottles of water use slogans like "filtered," "pure," "crystal clear," or "fresh," but plastic bottles still leach toxins. Not to mention they typically take petroleum to produce and are a blight to our landfills and oceans once they are discarded. Skip them and buy a glass or uncoated metal re-useable bottle! (See more in the plastics section that follows.)

Whole home filtration systems are pricey, but they filter water to all sources in your home—even your showers, which can release toxins into your skin and even your lungs through the steam. A good carbon-based or reverse osmosis system will help a lot. It's a very worthy investment.

Remember, you are what you eat, breathe, touch... and drink!

Shower Filters

As I mentioned above, it is important to filter shower water, too, especially if you don't have a whole home filter. Your water supply has things like chlorine and chlorimide in it, both of which go airborne in the steam and absorb into your lungs and skin. Shower filters are smart investments for your health. Most are carbon-based, which does a decent job. You can also find models that have a vitamin C filter, which does a better job at filtering out chlorimide than carbon does.

Get Rid of the Plastics! Especially Related to Food

There are many known toxins found in the plastic products we use and are exposed to everyday. Those associated with food and direct body exposure are particularly worrisome, as chemicals in these products can leach out into our food, beverages, and skin, and are easily stored in the body where they can do significant damage over the long term. These toxins include formaldehyde, phthalates, BPA, and toxic flame retardants, to name just a few. When stored in the body, they have been linked to increased risk of obesity, infertility, endocrine disruption, asthma, heart disease, and cancer.

A recent study released by Environmental Health Perspectives showed that most plastic products, from sippy cups to food wraps and water bottles, can release chemicals that act like the sex hormone estrogen. Yikes! This is of course not what most of us want our babies exposed to— they are too young to have the levels that can be exposed to them. The rest of us don't need additional exposure either. Excessive estrogen can lead to some of the diseases listed above.

It's easy enough to reduce some of our exposure, even in a plastic-filled world. Knowing that some things are unavoidable, consider the following tips.

Avoid Heat: Plastics are known to leach out trace chemicals, especially when heated. Don't use plastic to reheat food. When using a microwave, especially avoid plastic and plastic-coated take-out containers! By the way, most take-out containers are now coated in plastics, even when the outside looks like paper, so be mindful. When you go to your favorite coffee chain to get that piping hot coffee, be aware that the take-out cups are almost always lined with plastics. Yikes, indeed! You might bring your own plastic-free travel mug or cup and ask your barista to make your order in it, or you could save money in the long run and buy a nice coffee maker or espresso machine to make your own at home. And, how many times have you left that plastic water bottle in the hot car for days (or weeks)? Did it taste a little funny when you took a sip? Yup, those are likely various leached toxic "plasticides." At least you don't have to worry about storage or shipping of the water cases to stores. I'm sure they air-condition all those semi-trucks that deliver the water bottles in the scorching summer heat. Right?! (Not likely.)

Drink Liquids out of Glass, Ceramic, Uncoated Metal, or Another Less Toxic Material. If you like to carry a water bottle, consider one of these alternatives. I try to always keep one with me to avoid plastic water bottles. My favorite is glass that has a silicone cover around it to protect it from breaking.

Silicone is a Better Replacement. Silicone is a natural substance that is believed to be safer for food and beverages. If you like to buy plastic-coated products, especially cooking utensils, consider swapping them out for heat-resistant, food grade silicone.

Use Glass for Food Storage. Glass containers are much better than plastic. The glass doesn't really have anything that will leach into your food. I use the Pyrex style glass storage containers. They last and I can safely microwave with them. For some bulky items, like my washed leafy greens, I use Ziploc bags but line them with unbleached, recycled paper towels first to minimize exposure to the plastic.

Buy Food Staples Stored in Glass Instead of Plastic. I buy most of my staple items, like mayonnaise, drinks, and so on in glass jars as often as possible. There are plenty of good options, though they are available less and less as we seem to be shifting to plastic containers. ☹

Skip the Receipts! Almost all receipts are now printed on thermal papers that are lined with BPA and other harmful chemicals. Research has shown even touching these can cause things like BPA to leach into your skin. If you don't need it, ask them not to print or to toss it for you.

Baby Products: Keep the plastics away from your kids! Use glass bottles with silicone nipples. Find sippy cup alternatives, and be mindful of all the plastic toys they shove straight into their mouths. The stuffed animals typically come with chemical by-products in the fabrics from production too, so wash them well before letting your kids play with them, or find good organic sourced alternatives.

Metal Cans are Coated in Plastic. Almost all metal cans that store foods in the grocery store (e.g., tomato sauce, beans, soups) are lined with plastic coating. Instead, you can either prepare whole foods or look for glass jars when available.

BPA Alternatives May Not be Any Better. I always look for non-BPA products. That being said, there is emerging data that shows the alternatives may not be much better. The jury is still out, but it is best to be cautious and avoid plastic as much as possible. Even without BPA, they can still leak other toxins like phthalates.

Microplastics: There is also a big systemic problems with microplastics. These measure at 5mm or smaller and come from all kinds of plastic sources, including: waste, cosmetics, foods (from packaging, but also soil and water contamination), clothing, air and more. They can easily get into our bodies. In fact, research has estimated that the average person can get between 74,000 and 120,000 particles in their body a year. Yikes! The more we all move away from plastics as heavily as we use them now, the better.

Nonstick Cookware is Not as Safe as Proclaimed

Nonstick cookware has problems similar to plastics. While handy, the substances used to make nonstick cookware have been shown to also give off toxins that are not good for us, and they pollute our water supplies and environment. There are some toxins that are released from cooking with non-stick cookware on too high a heat. These noxious gases, when released, are particularly potent and problematic. But even at so-called "proper temperatures," nonstick cookware can create problems, leaching chemicals into your foods as they cook, or if you accidentally scrape off some of the material when stirring.

Animal studies have shown that the base chemicals used to make Teflon—one of the most commonly used nonstick materials—can cause growth defects, cancer, liver damage, immune system damage, and have even caused death in lab rats and monkeys. An EPA advisory panel reports it as a "likely carcinogen" in humans.

One type of nonstick coating that looks encouraging is made by a company called Scanpan. They make a full line of pans that uses a whole new coating technique that they call GreenTek, which allows them to bond the nonstick surface without using the noxious chemicals known to be of greatest concern. Their classic line uses a titanium ceramic surface that can even withstand metal cooking utensils. They are made from 100% recycled materials.

While Scanpan looks promising, we know what the best non-toxic materials are, they include: stainless steel, enamel, ceramic, glass, and cast iron. These are non-toxic options that should be your main staples for cooking. A little olive or avocado oil at medium heat will do just fine to help lubricate the pans for food!

General Resource Guide for Your Home

One fantastic resource for general home needs is the EWG's Healthy Living Home Guide, which includes more than twenty different types of products for building, making improvements, and furnishing your home. You'll find quick, inexpensive changes you can make, as well as bigger changes and investments you can take on when building, remodeling, or redecorating. Categories include:

- Air
- Carpet
- Cleaners and Air Fresheners
- Lights
- Mattresses
- Paint
- Reducing Household Dust
- Upholstered Furniture
- Wood Stains and Finishes
- And more…

Find the guide at www.ewg.org/healthyhomeguide.

Sunlight Nutrients: *Why you Need to Make Sure to Get Enough Light for Good Health*

Sunlight gets a bad rap. While it is true that too much exposure to ultraviolet (UV) spectrum light can be damaging, the same can be true for too little exposure to the many types of light waves that are essential nutrients. A growing field of health experts now believe we have overcompensated and now have too little exposure, which is having damaging consequences. There is research to back it up.

Sun exposure is a critical contributor to a number of health-related functions. Our bodies' largest organ, the skin, absorbs these nutrients and feeds our cells in key ways. Production of vitamin D is one of many examples that is well known. Sunlight is also key to regulating our circadian rhythm, which partly controls sleep quality. Even the infrared, red, and other invisible parts of the light spectrum are critical for the health of our *mitochondria*, for producing collagen, and many other key functions. (Mitochondria are the powerhouse of our cells and the strongest link to longevity.)

In a new world obsessed with sunscreen, UV-blocking windows, and sunglasses, we might be at the point of keeping ourselves too limited from its benefits.

Vitamin D

By now most of us know about the importance of having enough vitamin D in our body. It is critical for bone health, gut health, immune function, mood, and other metabolic functions, and yet experts believe many of us are chronically low in this nutrient. The primary way we get Vitamin D is through sunlight exposure and/or supplementation (Vitamin D3 is the form you want in supplements, by the way). It is not readily available in most natural foods.

For most fair-skinned people, it only takes about ten to fifteen minutes of exposure a day, without sunscreen, to get good amounts of vitamin D. Darker-skinned people need more sun exposure, as melanin in the skin slows down vitamin D production. The sun isn't high enough in the sky at all hours of the day to give us what we need for our vitamin D intake. Midday sun is ideal, and late spring to early fall is the best time to get optimal sun exposure. But worry not, with proper exposure you can bank up enough to get you through the leaner months. That said, it is always a good idea to get your vitamin D levels checked to make sure you are getting enough. And if you have skin issues, like skin cancers or basal cell carcinoma, etc., it is important to check with your doctor.

There are some great apps for smartphones to help determine your ideal sun exposure and to give you tips for reaching this ideal. I use the dminder app. It's available for both Apple and Android devices at http://bit.ly/2Q9gpEi. You can learn more about vitamin D deficiency at http://bit.ly/38v8Y2r.

Circadian Rhythm

If you have trouble sleeping, you might have been told to try a melatonin supplement. The reason this has become a popular sleep remedy is because of sunlight's impact on our circadian rhythm, which is critical for positive sleep function.

Put simply, sunlight triggers the production of melatonin when your eyes are exposed. This is hugely important for your circadian rhythm, which helps regulate your sleep and alertness cycles. We evolved for millions of years in carefully synched rhythm with sunlight exposure. In the modern world, our sun-deprived and increased exposure to fake lighting are now understood to be messing up that rhythm.

Because most of us work in offices without the full light spectrum of the sun (modern bulbs only have a partial light spectrum), we are not getting the right quantities or quality of light. We are also flooded with too much blue light from fluorescent and LED sources, including computer screens and smartphones.

One quick and easy thing to do for our circadian rhythm is to go out in the sun, even if just for a few minutes each morning when we wake up, to kickstart our cycle. That won't fully do the trick, but it helps.

Another trick is to soften your lights in the evening. If you have dimmers, use them. Otherwise, turn off non-essential lights and start to prepare your body for sleep at least a couple of hours before going to bed. Imagine that at night, when we were evolving in pre-industrial times, we would have had only the camp fire, candlelight, or other soft lighting after sundown.

You can also install *blue blockers* on your computer and smartphone. Blue light is the part of the spectrum we don't want much exposure to in the evening. There are some smart apps that will automatically adjust your screens throughout the day, and especially in the evening, so that its colors match nature more. The paid app Iris (www.iristech.co) is available for most devices and the free app f.lux (www.justgetflux.com) is available for Mac computers. Windows 10 apparently has its own blue light blocker baked in, but Google "blue light blocker apps for computer monitors" for other options for PCs. Apple iOS has a "nightshift" mode that will adjust away from blue light in the evenings. Make sure to turn it on in your settings! Android phones can try the Twilight: Blue Light Filter app. You can also dim your monitors and screens in the evening and try to avoid any computer usage before bedtime.

There are also numerous companies that make blue-light-blocking glasses. Dave Asprey has written extensively on this. Learn more here: http://bit.ly/2ENFn5O.

The Incredible Healing Powers of Infrared and Red-Light Spectrums

Red light and infrared light are two beneficial spectrums of light that we get from the sun when we have enough exposure. These are well-studied types of light that have shown many benefits in clinical trials. They have been proven to boost your mitochondria and energy levels, grow more collagen, heal skin, get your *lymph* (a fluid containing white blood cells) flowing better, boost the immune system, reduce inflammation (including arthritis), and open up your detox pathways.

Through my studies, I'd known about the benefits of the infrared light spectrum for many years. On the recommendation of my Functional Medicine doctor, about two years prior to writing this, I finally started going to a local spa and doing infrared saunas three times a week. My doctor wanted me to do this primarily for the detox benefits. Research has shown that infrared light not only helps you detox by making you sweat, but the invisible rays also penetrate deeper into your body and stimulate your cells to release stored toxins.

I also wanted to go because I knew of the anti-inflammatory effects it can have on the body, including pain reduction.

After twenty-plus years of back pain, I had an MRI a few years ago that showed I have at least six bulging disks in my back. I was really looking for solutions to ease the daily pain. I had tried seemingly everything over the past twenty years to help ease my back pain. Most of it hadn't worked (sorry, chiropractors who took thousands of my dollars). The only things that had worked were daily yoga, some help from a physical therapist, and now infrared and red-light therapy.

I went to the infrared sauna faithfully for about seven months, and I found it to be very helpful. I can't attest to its detox capacities, but it helped my back pain significantly. I experienced about a forty to fifty percent reduction in pain, which really excited me.

After a while it became challenging to get to the spa as often, so I considered purchasing an infrared sauna for my home. That's when I came across a device called the Joovv. The company sells a combination of infrared and red-light rays all in one device. It hangs on any door in your house, and you stand in front of it for ten to twenty minutes a day. I decided to give it a try as it was smaller and more affordable than a sauna. Plus they had a two-month trial window.

I was thrilled to learn that in just a couple of weeks, it worked as well on my back pain as the infrared sauna had, and after a month, improved it even further. (To be fair, I was using the Joovv almost every day versus the sauna, which was three times per week, so the sauna might have done just as well had I used it more.) After using it now for a year and a half, I can safely say I've had about a sixty-percent improvement in back pain symptoms.

For the longest time, I couldn't even sit for more than fifteen to twenty minutes. I'd get so uncomfortable. Sometimes my back would even "go out," and I could barely move for days. I have not had one big "back out" spell since starting it, and adding in my infrared/Joovv therapy is the only factor I have changed! They have published research on much of the benefits on their website, which I have read.

Red-light and infrared therapy have been life changers. I'd almost say they are miraculous. I encourage anyone to try it out. You can see if any local spas have these devices and try them out, or try out your own personal device. A few good brands I've heard of are: Sunlighten and Clearlight for infrared saunas, and Joovv and PlatinumLED for red-light/infrared combos. While all these are pricey, many companies have payment plans. What's more, you can think of this expense as a strong investment for your health and well-being.

If you decide you want to explore a device, make sure to get one powerful enough. There are many on the market that don't have the oomph you need for it to penetrate well or the right spectrum of light frequency.

Don't be so scared of the sun! Bottom line, at the bare minimum, consider ten to twenty minutes in the sun without sunscreen or sunglasses for as many days as you can in the seasons that allow for it. You don't want to overdo it, but underdoing it can also do harm. We evolved under the sun, and just like almost every other living species, we rely on it for more than warmth. There are numerous ways that it literally feeds us. But as always, you should follow the advice of your doctor.

Movement and Exercise: *Keep Yourself Moving to Maximize Vitality and Strength*

I'm sure most of you are aware that you need to engage in physical activity for good health. Because of that, I'm not going to cover it too deeply in this book, but I want to give a few pointers.

Being in good physical fitness has so many benefits. It improves your metabolism, strengthens bones, helps increase your insulin sensitivity and regulate blood sugar, improves sleep, and burns off stress chemicals just to name a few. Most importantly, though, getting adequate amounts of exercise can extend your lifespan.

In terms of exercise, pretty much every little thing you do helps. You don't have to train for a triathlon to get the benefits. Brisk walks, walking the dog, a hike, even cleaning the house, all of these activities help. Focus on movement! Don't let yourself get overwhelmed by what you think you should be doing at the expense of what you can do.

In fact, too much exercise or exercise that is too vigorous can do damage to the body, and we're not just talking about your muscles and joints. For starters, it can also tax your energy systems, your adrenal glands, and your mitochondria. If you aren't well, especially with regard to your overall energy capacity, then step into exercise slowly and thoughtfully. Let it energize you, not deplete you.

The following are a couple of ways to work more movement into your daily life. As always, consult with your physician before stating an exercise regimen.

For a more in-depth overview of the benefits of exercise, visit http://bit.ly/2OP1hXX.

Yoga

I've been talking about yoga throughout the book, but it bears repeating. I've been practicing yoga for more than twenty years. In that time, it's become an integral and extremely beneficial part of my life. I cannot speak highly enough the benefit it has been to me and how much I rely on it for grounding myself and tuning into what my body has to tell me.

There are three main benefits to yoga. First, you get a good physical workout and strengthening activity; second, it affords a good space to practice breathing deeply and calm your nervous system; and finally, it's great for stretching. For many it is also a spiritual practice.

When done right, it can be a powerful mindfulness practice. If I'm feeling particularly stressed or overly anxious, fifteen or twenty minutes can really help calm my system down. I also use it to help ease my back pain. Yoga helps open up my body, my joints, and my muscles.

Standing/Treadmill Desks, Exercise Balls as Chairs, and Other Tools for Staying in Motion at Work

Research shows that sitting all day at an office is one of the worst things we can do to our physical bodies. We did not evolve to be so inactive or to sit in such positions all day, which can slow our metabolism down to a crawl.

There are some things you can do in an office job to help. These methods not only help your body stay in better shape, they are also proven to boost mental clarity and alertness, which most of us could use more of!

Using a standing desk has been shown to be a vast improvement to sitting. You can get a tall desk or a topper that allows the workspace to rise. Veridesk is a quality brand, but there are many others now. Uplift is a company that offers motorized desks that rise up and down to your desires. I have one and love it. You can even add what is called a "motion board" or "motion stool" to help you increase activity.

I use a treadmill desk much of the time. By this I mean that I invested in a flat treadmill that goes under my tall standing desk. On a good day I can get in three to five miles of walking while I work. You might think it would be hard to work on a computer while walking on a treadmill, but I adjusted quickly to using a keyboard and mouse. I even have phone meetings while walking. No one can tell I'm on it! (Video calls are another matter.)

If your office requires you to sit, know that there are innovative companies that make under-desk elliptical and bike-pedaling devices. You can get some movement in all day while doing your work tasks. When I sit, I use a big exercise ball to sit on. It makes you put a little more effort into sitting up and balanced, plus you can bounce a little for motion and movement. It's also very comfortable when just sitting still. I've grown very used to it and don't even have a chair anymore.

Another good tip is to have walking meetings when possible. You can do this on the phone or in person. Ask colleagues to walk around outside or in a park. Research actually shows that walking meetings increase productivity and creativity as well as build stronger rapport among the team.

A few simple squats are another great way to squeeze good aerobic exercise and strength building into your day. You can do squats at work, or even in the kitchen at home while you are cooking. YouTube has many videos showing how to properly do a squat.

The Healing Power of Sleep: *Cultivating a Better Sleep Rhythm for Optimal Energy and Continual Healing*

As I discussed earlier when talking about our bodies Circadian Rhythm, sleep is far more critical to our health than most people realize. Getting good-quality sleep is a core pillar to good health. The bad news? In the West, we are getting less sleep and less-quality sleep than in the past. This is having some negative consequences on our health.

Our brains are one of the most energy-intensive organs in the body. Sleep is when our brain does its primary detox work, releasing and cleansing the chemical byproducts from all of its daily activities. This happens for our whole body as well. We face a barrage of stressors every day, from personal stress to environmental toxins, to poor food choices. If we don't get adequate sleep, the toxic byproducts that linger can cause all kinds of problems for us and have downstream consequences on all of our body systems.

Research shows that most of us are supposed to get between seven and nine hours of sleep a night, with eight hours being a good number to aim for. There is a relation between lack of adequate sleep and a host of diseases, like heart disease, diabetes, stroke risk, weight gain, and obesity. Disease rates rise in people who get less than seven hours on average. Less-than-optimal sleep also impairs mental performance and increases one's risk of physical accidents.

To (over)simplify this, the process of how we get good sleep is significantly driven by both light exposure and hormones like melatonin and cortisol. Essentially, melatonin tells our body when to sleep and cortisol kicks in to help wake us and give us an energy boost to start our day. Our body systems are far more susceptible to not getting enough sleep when we get too much light too late in the evening, or poor-quality light at any point during the day. Light is one of the main factors that alerts the body to produce the correct hormones for sleeping and waking. As I shared earlier, these are all connected through what is called our circadian rhythm, which tells our body when it's time to sleep and wake. When our body system and all our hormones are off balance then our sleep gets thrown off as well.

Modern life is not synonymous with good sleep. Stress, poor-quality manmade light exposure, bad food choices or eating too late at night, noise, and lack of physical exercise, can all play a role in keeping us from properly sleeping.

How to Get Better Sleep

Make sure to get some exposure to sunlight first thing in the morning if you can. This helps set a proper circadian rhythm. You also want to keep lights dimmer in the evening, especially a couple of hours before bed. Remember, in nature, we only had maybe moonlight and a fire as we evolved for millions of years. This dimmer light alerted and trained our bodies, in fact our genes, that it was time to wind down.

If you are on your computer or watching bright TV with all the lights on in your house, your body will be disconnected from some of its natural alert mechanisms. Speaking of screens, as I said earlier, your smartphone, computer, and TV give off an inordinate amount of blue light, which in nature is not readily found at night. Avoid them before bed, and for your devices, get "blue blocking" software. See the previous Circadian Rhythm section for more tips.

Late-night snacking can screw up your sleep patterns as well, so make sure to stop eating about two hours or more before bed.

Learn more tips for good sleep health here: http://bit.ly/3vilgF9.

Our Collective Needs: *Building Resilient Community and Working for Social Change*

We have mostly discussed issues so far that are individually focused in terms of how to address them. Collective, societal and ecological issues have tremendous impact on us too, and we to them. Hopefully it has become clear in reading this book that there are a lot of bigger picture social and even political issues that are driving health challenges on our planet, from environmental degradation, rampant toxin exposure, lack of good policies and regulations to prevent, subpar health care coverage, corporate greed and many others.

We can each better take our health, both physically and mentally, into our own hands. But there are so many factors that are out of our individual control which still have an impact on us.

It certainly behooves us as individuals to have many of these social obstacles transform. I also believe that it is our collective responsibility to step up and be active voices in making social change for the betterment, not only for ourselves, but also for all of humanity. I believe it is a part of our sacred responsibility as co-inhabitants of this planet. And if we really want to get well, then these issues must be addressed.

I believe we are all our sisters' and brothers' keepers. We need each other to thrive and I think we are ultimately only as strong as our weakest links. Human suffering has ripple effects just as toxic as the other things I mentioned throughout this book.

All of us are affected by what happens to our fellow man, certainly most acutely in our communities, but also around the globe. Example: that there are almost ninety-three million people living near poverty in America has direct consequences on all of us. People in poverty are sicker, tend to be more connected to crime, and need higher levels of social support. If we don't work to pull these people out of poverty and despair, we will pay far more over time as the costs of trying to manage so many of these after-effects far outweigh what we would spend on prevention.

And money is the least of it. We are witnessing the unraveling of our social fabric, evidenced by things like the rapid rise in mass shootings, even school shootings. Millions live in fear for their lives everyday, from violence inside and outside their homes. The growingly toxic political discourse is another example, as well as so many other societal ills. The climate crises will also have tremendous impacts on our health and happiness.

I don't mean to sound overly dour. We are seeing a lot of positive progress too that we should champion and be proud of, but far too many of us are sitting on the sidelines of social change work and woefully undereducated about what is happening on our planet. Too many see politics as a dirty game, but our government quite simply is how we organize ourselves. If we don't like how we are being organized, we must get deeply educated and engage in pushing it in a direction that would serve our highest potential and needs.

My friend and a mentor, Marianne Williamson, I think says it best in her profound book, *A Politics of Love*:

Democracy gives us rights, but it also gives us responsibilities, not just to receive the blessings of liberty but to tend to them in our time and bequeath them to our children. This is not a job for someone else. It's a job for each of us. We the people are the only true guardians of democracy. We have a much greater purpose on earth than to just get what we want. That has always been America's greatness: that we stood for something higher than ourselves and strove for something higher than ourselves. Until we retrieve that greatness, we will continue to go down. But as soon as we do retrieve it, we will miraculously rise up again. For on the level of spirit we have wings.

Let's look at a few more specifics. In the United States, our healthcare system leaves far too many people behind. Even those that have decent healthcare can struggle to cover all their costs. And what about prevention care? Most insurance companies do not cover much. We wait until someone is already sick to provide supports (if even then). By then it's far more expensive and sometimes too late. We need nutritionists, health coaches, exercise support, longer doctors office visits, much better research funding and expanded scope, and many more improvements and supports.

Mental health as well. As we discussed, stress, trauma and emotional issues are one of the biggest drivers of disease, and yet very few people have coverage for mental health. It's out of reach for far too many. It's not just disease we are seeing manifest from these gaps, it's also violence, crime and despair.

We need to make sure we are tending to our most vulnerable. The effects of trauma and PTSD are real and rampant. **Studies show that millions of our children who live in our more violent communities suffer the same kind of PTSD as vets returning from war.** Let that soak in for a minute. They live with the constant threat of violence that can quickly degrade emotional health and lead to lifelong consequences. We know how to better address these issues. There are many experts and practitioners who have methods to help turn this around, but funding is minimal even though we pay far less on prevention and smart interventions that we engage in than after problems already emerge.

We need more social wrap around services in our cities. We need Conflict Resolution Education, Social and Emotional Learning and Restorative Justice in schools, as well as well as things like mindfulness and mediation programs—all of which have already proven to help positively change the whole climate of a school and turn lives around. It also sets these kids up for far more productive and happy adult lives.

Not to mention our food policies are also outdated and counterproductive. We subsidize things like processed grains and high fructose corn syrup, for example, rather than the more nutritious options described in this book. People often can't afford organic foods, or other whole foods and healthier options, when the cheap and fast versions are artificially propped up by our tax dollars. Our FDA is underfunded and too often aligned with corporate interests rather than social wellbeing. We need more funding on food and nutrition research, from independent third parties instead of the big food companies whose primary objective is profit, not real health.

We allow far too many toxins into our environment. Why do we allow so many poisons to leach out in every direction? Because there are powerful interests who make a profit off of them and because we don't have the political will to invest in cleaner alternatives.

The average America is asleep at the wheel. Too many politicians may be bought and paid for by their big donors, which they need to win elections. Big money has undue influence there. But we are still the people who vote. That is something that has more power than anything else. Voting is important, but so is speaking up and making sure our elected officials know what we want them to be putting their attention on in order to earn our votes—citizen lobbying.

It is critical that we all stand up and engage in using our power for not only our own good, but for the good of all. We far too often abandon each other. That is not the kind of ground from which to have fertile communities, where we can feel nourished, safe and with the ability to live vibrant, happy lives. We must step into our power and invest at least some of our time in pushing for these kinds of changes. The consequences of not doing so are too dire. For ourselves and for our fellow man.

Once again, I think Marianne Williamson says it beautifully in her book *A Politics of Love*:

Something is rising up from the depths today, centered not in any one geographical area, ethnic identity, or national identity. It's the evolutionary lure of a sustainable future, calling us to remember who we really are and inviting us to rise up from the past. It is a hunger felt among all the people of the world. We are stirred to live our lives in a different way; to align ourselves with something truer and deeper than mere bricks and mortar or dollars and cents. This stirring brings with it a deeper reverence, for earth and sky, and for each other. If we truly want a different world, we must be willing to think in a different way and live in a different way than we do now.

Indeed. And it's to all our benefit when we do. Your health depends on this as much as anything else. May we all step into a new level of co-creation for the kind of world we all long for. It will be ours when we create it.

In Conclusion...

I hope the resources within this book have proven helpful. I'm beyond grateful that you decided to take the time with me to explore this important information with me. It's all a guide to a healthier, more vibrant life.

There are many choices within this book that you might take on, but don't let the long list of possible changes overwhelm you. Start with the four pillars in the first half of the book, begin to integrate dietary changes into your life, and then pick and choose from the rest as you are able. Every step you take should lead to improvements.

Hopefully, as you begin to feel the shifts in your health and well-being, you will be more positively engaged in this life of yours and become an even bigger blessing to all those around you. Maybe you'll even inspire a few folks to join you.

If you do feel inspired by this book, I'd love to hear from you. Share your personal and nutritional journey with me on my Facebook at:
www.facebook.com/MatthewAlbracht
or write me at: info@nourishyourselfwhole.com.

Also, if you loved the book and have a bit of time to spare, I would really appreciate a short review on Amazon as it would help new readers find my book.

I also take coaching clients as I'm able if you would like a little more one-on-one support. You can find further information on that and additional and ongoingly updated resources on my website at:

www.nourishyourselfwhole.com.
May you continue to discover and embrace good health for a joyful and vibrant life!

Nourish Your Self Whole

Additional Resources:

Informational Websites:

SELF Nutrition Data: This is one of my favorite websites to learn about the nutrition content of various foods. You'll find detailed nutrition information for fresh and processed foods. www. nutritiondata.self.com

Chris Kresser: One of my favorite teachers and Functional Medicine practitioners. Chris has loads of good, well researched information on his website—especially around nutrition.
www. chriskresser.com

Dr. Mark Hyman: One of the leaders in the field of Functional Medicine and nutrition. He is also an expert on fat, sugar and other key health issues. His site has a lot of good information. www. drhyman.com

The Institute for Functional Medicine: Functional Medicine determines how and why illness occurs and restores health by addressing the root causes of disease for each individual. IFM helps trains doctors and practitioners in Functional Medicine and they have certifications and listings of practitioners around the nation on their website. www.ifm.org

Functional Medicine Coaching Academy: Find certified health coaches through this service (or train to become a health coach yourself).
www.directory.functionalmedicinecoaching.org

MindBodyGreen: Provides a nice variety of articles on health and wellness related topics.
www.mindbodygreen.com

EWG (Environmental Working Group): A fantastic organization and resource. They have rankings of thousands of food and health related products, grade their ingredients—looking for pesticides, toxins, and irritants. Check out their consumer guide. They also have great smartphone apps that allow you to scan product barcodes through your smartphone's camera and it tells you how products and foods rank on their health ratings scale.
www.ewg.org

Peter Attia's Eating Academy: Excellent research and writing on a range of topics, including Cholesterol. www.peterattiamd.com

Vegan Resources: Kris Carr is great if you are looking for good vegan health food resources, here is a good site. www.kriscarr.com Another great site is the Food Revolution Network, from Ocean and John Robbins. www.foodrevolution.org

Center for Nonviolent Communication: A global organization that supports the learning and sharing of Nonviolent Communication (NVC), and helps people peacefully and effectively resolve conflicts in personal, organizational, and political settings. www.cnvc.org

Multidisciplinary Association for Psychedelic Studies (MAPS): a non-profit research and educational organization that develops medical, legal, and cultural contexts for people to benefit from the careful uses of psychedelics, particularly for PTSD and psychological healing purposes. www.maps.org

Books

Nutrition

The Paleo Cure: Prevent and Reverse Disease, Lose Weight Effortlessly, and Look and Feel Better than Ever by Chris Kresser

Food: What the Heck Should I Eat? (Paperback title is *Food: WTF Should I Eat*) by Mark Hyman, M.D

Paleo Principles: The Science Behind the Paleo Template, Step-by-Step Guides, Meal Plans, and 200+Healthy and Delicious Recipes for Real Life. By Sarah Ballantyne, PhD

Deep Nutrition by Catherine Shanahan, MD

Eating on the Wild Side: The Missing Link to Optimum Health by Jo Robinson

Recipes

Nom Nom Paleo: Food for Humans (Volume 1) by Michelle Tam and Henry Fong

Food: What the Heck Should I Cook?: More than 100 Delicious Recipes—Pegan, Vegan, Paleo, Gluten-free, Dairy-free, and More—For Lifelong Health by Mark Hyman

Paleo Leap: A website with gobs of free health conscious recipes. www.paleoleap.com/paleo-diet-recipes

Functional Medicine and Deeper Healing

The Immune System Recovery Plan: A Doctor's 4-Step Program to Treat Autoimmune Disease by Susan Blum, MD, MPH

The Disease Delusion: Conquering the Causes of Chronic Illness for a Healthier, Longer, and Happier Life by Dr. Jeffrey S. Bland

Gut and Psychology Syndrome: Natural Treatment for Autism, Dyspraxia, A.D.D., Dyslexia, A.D.H.D., Depression, Schizophrenia Revised & enlarged Edition by Natasha Campbell-McBride (This book suggestion is for people with serious gut problems only.)

The Whole30: The 30-Day Guide to Total Health and Food Freedom by Hartwig Urban, Melissa and Dallas Hartwig

Pets!

Canine Nutrigenomics: The New Science of Feeding Your Dog for Optimum Health by W. Jean Dodds and Diana R. Laverdure

Psychology/Spirit/Social Change

A Return to Love; Healing the Soul of America; and A Politics of Love by Marianne Williamson (three different books)

The Untethered Soul by Michael A. Singer

The Power of Attachment: How to Create Deep and Lasting Intimate Relationships by Diane Poole Heller, PhD

The Body Keeps the Score: Brain, Mind, and Body in the Healing of Trauma by Bessel Van der Kolk MD

Wired for Love: How Understanding Your Partner's Brain and Attachment Style Can Help You Defuse Conflict and Build a Secure Relationship by Stan Tatkin, PsyD, MFT

Hardwiring Happiness: The New Brain Science of Contentment, Calm and Confidence by Rick Hanson, PhD

Coming Back to Life: Practices to Reconnect our Life, Our World by Joanna Macey and Molly Young Brown

A New Earth by Eckhart Tolle

Food Fix: How to Save Our Health, Our Economy, Our Communities, and Our Planet--One Bite at a Time by Mark Hyman, MD

Drawdown: The Most Comprehensive Plan Ever Proposed to Reverse Global Warming by Paul Hawken and Tom Steyer

Podcasts

The Whole View, Modern Science and A Real Life Approach to Health: Sarah Ballantyne PhD (scientist) and Stacy Toth humorously talk about paleo lifestyle.

Revolution Health Radio: Chris Kresser's Podcast. He's one of my favorite experts in Functional Medicine.

The Doctors Farmacy: Mark Hyman, MD

The Healthy Rebellion Radio Podcast: With Robb Wolf focuses on Paleo diet, nutrition, fitness and health.

Nourish Balance Thrive: These guys are smart. Lot's of good topics. Often more related to fitness, but still broad enough for those for whom that isn't their focus.

Conversations the Matter: Marianne Williamson.

The Tim Ferriss Show: Features a variety of topics and guests, often related to personal growth and health.

Super Soul Sunday: Oprah's interviews turned into a podcast.

Printable Cheat Sheet Shopping List

Remember that you can download a handy ***Printable Cheat Sheet Shopping List*** I created just for readers of this book, with key lists and tips included in my tips sections for each of the four pillars. Just print it out to take with you, or save the .pdf to your smartphone so you always have it. Visit: www.nourishyourselfwhole.com/printable-cheat-sheet

Favorite Foods Shopping List

You can find a list of many of my favorite foods and especially healthier replacements for many favorite staples on my website at:

www.nourishyourselfwhole.com/resources

Check my site as I update these resources regularly. www.nourishyourselfwhole.com/resources

Activism and Social Change Organizations

Just a few, related to issues addressed in this book.

The Peace Alliance: A great org that advocates for peacebuilding and practical policies we can implement to bring about more peace and connection in society. They have a Blueprint for Peace that focuses on: humanizing justice systems; empowering community interventions; teaching peace in our schools; enhancing personal and interpersonal supports; and fostering international peacebuilding initiatives. I'm also a co-founder. www.peacealliance.org

Nutrition Coalition: They have a primary goal of ensuring that U.S. nutrition policy is based on rigorous scientific evidence, ensuring evidence-based nutrition policy. www.nutritioncoalition.us

Alliance for Natural Health: The largest organization in the US and abroad working to protect your right to utilize safe, effective, and inexpensive healing therapies based on high-tech testing, diet, supplements, and lifestyle changes. They believe a system that is single-mindedly focused on "treating" sick people with expensive drugs, rather than maintaining healthy people, is neither practical nor economically sustainable. www.anh-usa.org

Pachamama Alliance: A global community that offers people the chance to learn, connect, engage, travel and cherish life for the purpose of creating a sustainable future that works for all. Particularly focused on ecology and environmental issues. www.pachamama.org

River Phoenix Center for Peacebuilding: Their mission is to enrich the lives of individuals, families, and communities by providing and promoting the best practices and principles of peacebuilding and global sustainability.
www.centerforpeacebuilding.org

Bibliography/Notes

On my website, you will find a bibliography of key citations, along with relevant notes linking to informative articles on topics I share in this book. If you want to dig deeper into research on some of the key topics I cover in this book, or read informative articles to explore issues further, you will find a fair amount on my website at: www.nourishyourselfwhole.com/book-bibliography

Nourish Your Self Whole

Acknowledgements

My eternal gratitude and love to Rob Ablon. Not only is your partnership and support invaluable to me on a personal level, but you helped me so much throughout this project, with great ideas and insights (especially helping come up with the title!). I am beyond blessed to have you in my life and looking forward to where the journey continues to lead us.

Thank you to a great editor, Jessica Hatch, who gave much invaluable feedback and guidance. Also Daniel Johnson for the proofread and additional edits.

Many thanks to Heather MacMillan, who has been a great coach through this whole process. For helping me to stay on target, giving me great input, edits and insights and for being a lovely person all around! Your help and support made this an even more empowering experience.

For my friends and loved ones who read parts of it early on and gave me important encouragement, feedback and editing suggestions. Particularly Julie Hess, Molly Albracht Sierra, Betsy Dee, Gia Calvillo, Nancy Wright Maxwell, Debbie Urban, Dana Santa Cruz, and others! You know who you are.

To my awesome Mom and Dad who have positively encouraged this book (and my life) the whole way. Grateful to my entire family for so much love and inspiration. I hope the information within feeds and nourishes you as you have me.

To Marianne Williamson, from whom many of my sensibilities and writing skills have arisen through working (and writing) with you. I feel honored to have been able to learn so much from you over the years. Your love and support have meant so much.

To my Functional Medicine doc, Dr. Stephanie Daniel, for working closely with me these last few years and helping me figure out the best path to health. I've made great strides!

Finally, to all the other people who have helped me along my journey. Astraea in particular, thank you for the guidance, patience and great care—I can feel myself evolving! There are too many others to list without getting myself into trouble for missing someone. I wouldn't be the man I am without an inspiring and loving community of people who helped nurture me along the journey. And what a journey indeed!

About Matthew

Matthew Albracht currently lives in Oakland, CA with his loving partner Rob and amazing Golden Retriever, Cooper.

He is a social changemaker, wellness coach and advocate. His writings have appeared on CNN, HuffPost, Medium and other outlets. He experienced significant health improvements in 2015 that changed the course of his life. They were born from nutritional changes he discovered and implemented. He now devotes much of his time towards functional nutrition and wellness education and advocacy. He is a Functional Medicine Certified Health Coach (FMCHC) through the Functional Medicine Coaching Academy.

Matthew has a BA in psychology from Sonoma State University and a MA in Humanities and Leadership with a focus on Culture, Ecology and Sustainable Community from New College of California.

He was formerly the Executive Director and is currently a Board Member of The Peace Alliance which advocates for domestic and international peacebuilding. (www.peacealliance.org)

www.NourishYourSelfWhole

Quick View Cheat Sheet Shopping Guide

The information below is a guide of healthier options for grocery shopping, as well as items to avoid. Also some fun replacement cheats to swap out for some favorite unhealthy foods.

Remember that you can also download this information as a .pdf entitled: ***Printable Cheat Sheet Shopping List***. Visit: www.nourishyourselfwhole.com/printable-cheat-sheet

Highlighted:

- **Sugars**
  - o Sugars to Avoid
  - o Good Sugar Alternatives
  - o Decent Sugar Substitutes
- **Carbohydrates**
  - o Good Alternatives to Refined Flour
  - o Good Pasta Alternatives
  - o Good Complex Carbs
- **Fats**
  - o Best Types of Fats & Oils to Use
  - o Fats & Oils to Avoid
  - o Fat Smoke Point
- **Vegetables & Fruit**
- **My Favorite Foods List**

Sugars to Avoid

Foods contain naturally occurring and added sugars. You want to watch and limit both, but added sugars are the most troubling as more and more processed and packaged foods contain them. Look at your labels for any packaged foods to make sure there aren't too many grams of sugar listed (anything over just a few is a lot).

Whether it's something you stock at home, or that is put into a packaged food, some of the big baddies to avoid are:

- Sugar (cane, powdered, brown, etc.)
- High-fructose corn syrup
- Dextrose
- Maltose
- Glucose
- Fructose
- Corn sweetener
- Honey (raw ok in small amounts)
- Corn syrup
- Sucrose
- Sorghum syrup
- Sorbitol
- Lactose
- Molasses
- Syrup
- Fruit juice concentrate
- Artificial sweeteners: NutraSweet, saccharine, aspartame, etc.

Good Sugar Alternatives:

When you have the occasional treat, there are some tasty but still somewhat healthier options to sweeten your food. Three of the best alternatives are:

- Stevia
- Monk fruit (Lakanto brand is most common)
- Allulose

These options contain no calories and won't spike your blood sugar. Monk fruit and allulose looks like and converts into recipes just like sugar, and have a pleasant, sweet flavor not too dissimilar to refined sugar. Stevia comes now in many brands, and some have much more of an aftertaste than others. Look for a whole-foods source that isn't overly processed for the best flavor and quality.

The jury isn't completely in on how these effect your body, but they are likely better than real sugars when used in moderation.

Just Ok Sugar Substitutes:

(Use sparingly)

- Coconut Sugar
- Maple Syrup
- Maple Sugar
- Raw Honey

Good Alternatives to Refined Flours:
All three of these are decent substitutes for refined wheat flour. They don't break down into glucose as much as standard choices and can be used for the occasional baking needs.
- Cassava flour
- Almond flour
- Coconut flour

Pasta Alternatives:
- Spiralized vegetable noodles (I like carrot and zucchini. Sweet potato, butternut squash, and beet noodles are good, too.)
- Spaghetti squash (makes a fantastic alternative for spaghetti noodles).
- Shirataki noodles (made from a Japanese yam that are tasty and closer to traditional pasta. The brand I'm most familiar with is called Miracle Noodles.)
- Almond flour pastas are also available in some markets, typically in freezer section, and are quite tasty for the occasional treat (Cappellos is the brand I like).
- Quinoa or lentil pastas (with these grain-based alternatives, keep it to a minimum).

Good Complex Carbs:
Starchy vegetables are a good substitute that can help fill the refined carb void.
Some of the best starchy vegetables are:
- Sweet potatoes & yams,
- Jicama,

- Squash (e.g., butternut, acorn, kabocha, delicata, pumpkin, spaghetti, etc.)
- Turnips & Beets,
- Red-skinned potatoes,
- Parsnips,
- Celery root,
- Plantains,
- Traditional russet potatoes are ok too, but try to mix other varieties of potato into your diet as russets can be harder on the digestive system than others.

Best Types of Fats and Oils to Use:

(Diversity is important, so mix it up and get a variety each day.)

- Olive Oil (always extra virgin, cold-pressed)
- Avocado Oil
- Coconut Oil (virgin)
- Tallow and Lard (from good sources, like grass-fed animals)
- Butter and Ghee (Clarified Butter) (grass-fed is best)
- Palm Oil (sustainably sourced)
- Smaller amounts of cold- or expeller-pressed, unrefined nut and seed oils, such as macadamia, walnut, and sesame. Flax, chia, and hemp are also considered to be decent sources.
- Full-Fat Dairy. For those that can tolerate dairy, this can be a good source. (Organic, grass-fed sources are best.)
- Quality, Grass-Fed Animal Fats.

Fats and Oils to Avoid:

(Almost all processed foods contain one form or another of these toxic fats, so watch out!)

- Canola
- Soy
- Corn
- Sunflower
- Safflower
- Cottonseed
- Grapeseed
- Sesame (unless used cold-pressed in things like salad dressing, but never in processed foods or to cook with)
- Margarine
- Most non-stick cooking sprays (some new companies are using avocado or coconut oils, which may be better)
- Anything labeled "Vegetable Oil," "Shortening," or with words "Hydrogenated" or "Trans Fat" on label.

Fat Smoke Points:

(When cooking with oils, you want to keep them below their smoke point. When they get past their smoke point, they start to form dangerous free radicals.)

- Avocado Oil 520°F
- Ghee 485°F
- Palm Oil 450°F
- Coconut Oil (expeller pressed, refined) 450°F
- Coconut Oil (extra virgin) 350°F

- Macadamia Nut Oil 390° F
- Beef Tallow 400°F
- Duck Fat 375°F
- Lard 370°F
- Olive Oil (extra virgin) 320° F
- Butter 350°F

Much of this data is from: John Barron, "Healthiest Cooking Oil Comparison Chart with Smoke Points and Omega-3 Fatty Acid Ratios." Baseline of Health Foundation. http://bit.ly/2DakQYT

Vegetables & Fruit

You really can't go wrong in this department. Most fruits and vegetables can be liberally eaten (with some moderation on fruit because of the higher sugar content). Get a wide variety of colors for a broad spectrum of vitamins, minerals, phytonutrients and antioxidants.

Fiber: Vegetables and Fruits Contain Some of the Best Kinds

Another great benefit of vegetables and fruits is the important fiber content. Fiber can help bulk up the stool, including detoxified "bad stuff" our body needs to flush out, and move everything through the intestines more efficiently. It also helps minimize blood sugar spikes by slowing sugar breakdown and absorption, it helps feed good gut bacteria that provide numerous benefits for our healthy functioning, and more. Great sources of soluble and insoluble fiber include:

- leafy, green vegetables;
- yams and sweet potatoes;
- carrots and other root vegetables;
- squash;
- fruits with an edible peel, like apples and pears;
- berries;
- seeds;
- nuts.

Going Organic

As much as you possibly can, buy organic. The pesticides, herbicides, and fertilizers that are used to help produce conventionally grown crops are shown to be particularly toxic to humans.

I realize it's not always possible to buy organic, especially depending on where you live. The Environmental Working Group (EWG) has done a great job of identifying the biggest "problem" fruits and vegetables on their annual "Dirty Dozen" list. They do rigorous testing and research to identify the most pesticide-ridden fruits and vegetables, the ones we should buy organic, every year.

Here are this year's Dirty Dozen, with the worst culprit first:

- Strawberries
- Spinach
- Nectarines
- Apples
- Grapes

- Peaches
- Cherries
- Pears
- Tomatoes
- Celery
- Potatoes
- Sweet Bell Peppers
- [Dis]honorable Mention: Hot Peppers.

Please note, this list can change a bit from year to year (though it tends to stay pretty consistent). Check www.ewg.org for the most recent list.

If you can't find fresh organic versions of these foods and you really need one of these items, consider looking for organic frozen.

Speaking of cleaner conventionally grown options, EWG also has a list called the "Clean Fifteen," listing the least contaminated. This year's includes:

- Avocados
- Sweet Corn
- Pineapples
- Cabbage
- Onions
- Sweet Peas (frozen)
- Papayas
- Asparagus
- Mangos
- Eggplant
- Honeydew Melon
- Kiwi

- Cantaloupe
- Cauliflower
- Broccoli

On a related note, EWG makes a great set of phone apps for identifying more and less toxic foods in general. You can also check out their food score website at www.ewg.org/foodscores. Here, they rank the health of food items you might find at the grocery store.

My Favorite brands of Staples and Treats:

There is a variety of items here that I enjoy. You can find updates and clickable links on my website at: www.nourishyourselfwhole.com/shopping-list

REFINED CARB ALTERNATIVES:

These lower glycemic load "carb" alternatives are all gluten free and won't wreak as much havoc on your body as many refined flours. You can bake with these or use them for a number of cooking needs. They taste great and are paleo friendly and gluten free. You should still be mindful about how much you indulge.

> **Paleo Pancake and Waffle Mix by Birch Benders:** This mix is sooo good. Totally hits my need for occasional pancakes, without the giant carb hit.

> **Cassava Flour by Otto's Naturals:** This flour is made from Yucca root. Another great alternative baking

flour that is a staple in low glycemic non-wheat flour baking.

Coconut Flour by Nutiva: This is a great alternate for baking.

Cassava and Coconut Flour Tortilla's by Siete: These taste good and are a great alternative for those that really want some kind of carb alternative for wraps or other uses.

Shirataki Noodles by Miracle Noodles: Made from a Japanese yam. These are zero carb and gluten free. Taste good. They have an assortment of styles, fettuccini, angel hair, etc.

Almond Flour by Bob's Red Mill: There are several types, all good. Super fine from blanched or non-blanched whole almonds. Other brands good as well.

SNACKS & APPETIZERS:

Mary's Crackers: These are gluten free and relatively clean ingredients if you want a crackery snack. They have many flavors. Crunchy and nice.

Siete Grain Free Tortilla Chips: These are AMAZING! So light and crispy. Tastes surprisingly like corn chips. They are made from Cassava and fried in Avocado oil. Both are better for you than other chips made with cheap industrial seed vegetable oils which are rancid and toxic.

Sweet Potato Chips or Blue Corn Chips: Jackson's Honest chips are fried in coconut oil, which is a far better option than cheap vegetable oils.

Coconut Almond Butter by Maranatha: This is so tasty! Creamy and delicious. A blend of almond butter with coconut cream. One of my favorite treats is a tablespoon of it.

Sardines by Wild Planet: These are a great snack. Loads of good omega 3 fats and decadent. I like to get the ones packed in extra virgin olive oil as they help protect the fat from the fish.

Roasted Seaweed by SeaSnax: This is one of the only seaweed snacks that uses olive oil to roast in, not a cheap, crappy oil like canola.

Meat Bars, Grassfed, by Epic: These are paleo friendly. I bring them with me when traveling and flying. Make a good jolt of nourishment.

Hummus, Organic by Hope: Make sure to get a brand that has good oils. Most use canola or other cheap, bad oils. Hope brand uses extra virgin olive oil.

SWEETENERS:

You don't have to fully give up your sweet tooth! These sweeteners are less negatively impactful as cane sugar or high fructose corn syrup.

Monkfruit Sweetener by Lakanto: Tastes good and makes a nice replacement for cane sugar. You can use it the same, cup for cup. This has almost no glycemic load (blood sugar raiser).

Stevia: Liquid or powdered packets: Avoid cheap crappy stevia's, they don't taste good. Only get 100% Stevia, not mixed with other types of junk sweetener. Just say NO to Truvia.

Raw Honey by YS: Be sure to buy raw honey, unfiltered if you can. Heat processing kills many of the good nutrients in honey.

Coconut Sugar, Organic, by Big Tree Farms: Nice flavor, works well for cooking. Occasional treat.

Maple Syrup, Organic by Coombs Family Farm: This should be used only occasionally, it still has a lot of sugar in it.

OILS AND FATS:

Olive Oil, Napa Valley Naturals Organic: Great flavor and good quality. Always buy cold pressed extra virgin.

Amphora Nueva Olive Oils: This is a great company that carefully sources its oils (and amazing flavored, barrel aged Balsamic Vinegars). Found online only. www.amphoranueva.com

Ghee, 4th and Heart Plain and Heart Pink Himalayan Sea Salt: Love these. Ghee is a great alternative for butter. Both of these are grassfed. Ghee has a high smoke point, so you can sauté with it at higher temperatures. I use the plain for cooking and the sea salt version for snacking.

Coconut Oil by Artisana: Nutiva brand is fine as well, it's more affordable, but I like Artisana's taste.

Avocado Oil: I use La Tourangelle for more delicate flavorful needs, like salad dressing. I use Primal Kitchen or Chosen Foods for cooking. Avocado oil has a high smoke point, and doesn't oxidize as easily. So you can sauté with it at higher temperatures. Or even for frying. Chosen foods makes a pan spray as well.

Avocado Oil Mayo: Primal Kitchen or Chosen Foods. Tasty and much better than almost all other mayo's, as they all use cheap, unhealthy vegetable oils.

Macadamia Nut Oil: by Roland. Mac oils are great for salad dressings.   Healthy oil, don't need a lot though, just a splash mixed in with olive and avocado. Another option is Piping Rock.

DAIRY ALTERNATIVES:

Coconut Milk, Simple, Native Forest: This is one of the only brands that makes it without Guar Gum, which can cause digestive problems for some people. This is a heavy coc0nut milk used primarily for cooking, not for a "milk" substitute for things like cereal.

Coconut Cashewmilk by Forager: This is in refrigerated sections only, but has very simple ingredients and also no gums. Tastes great if you can find it!

CoYo Coconut Yogurt: This coconut-based yogurt is very delightful and surprisingly creamy. It also makes a great substitute for sour cream, a similar consistency. Since it's refrigerated, it's at stores only.

HERBS, SPICES & FLAVORINGS:

Celtic Sea Salt

Himalayan Sea Salt

Real Salt, by Redmond: This "sea salt" comes from an ancient seabed in Utah that was not exposed to modern toxins like sea salts are often today. Another bonus is this is one of the only sea salts that has a decent amount of iodine.

Balsamic Vinegar: Amphora Nueva (online only) makes these barrel aged vinegars that really are pretty amazing. My favorites are the red "cinnamon & pear" and the white "apricot". These are slightly thicker and a touch of sweet. But it doesn't take much to flavor a great salad dressing or for a drizzle. www.amphoranueva.com

Swiss Chard Powder by Dr. Cowan's Garden: This delightful flavoring powder is nutrient dense. If you have a hard time squeezing in enough vegetables in a day, try this out. They also have Kale and number of other great options. I put a spoonful in salad dressings, sprinkle into soups, etc. Great way to spice up and packed with nutrients!

MISCELLANEOUS:

Bone Broth, Grassfed by Kettle and Fire or Epic: Great source of nutrients for your gut and skin health, plus so much more. Should be a dietary staple.

Wild Salmon by Wild Planet: These are a great alternative to tuna (which is high in mercury). Loads of good omega 3 fats.

Check my website as I update this list periodically as I find new stuff.
www.nourishyourselfwhole.com/shopping-list

Made in United States
Orlando, FL
20 May 2022

18046190R00171